P9-AGG-340

LIVE LONG, LIVE STRONG

An Integrative Approach to
Cancer Care and Prevention

To Your Health!

LIVE LONG, LIVE STRONG
An Integrative Approach to Cancer Care and Prevention

Dr. Mao Shing Ni, Ph.D., D.O.M., L.Ac.
and
Frances K. Lam, MATCM, L.Ac.

TAO OF
WELLNESS
PRESS

Dedication

To oncologist Lorne Feldman —it was your courage, inspiration and collaboration that was the genesis of this book. You urged me to share this information with the world so that there would be less suffering, and more health and belief in the Higher Power. I miss you!

I dedicate this book to the many patients who have shown me their courage when facing life-threatening diagnosis. Their determination to change their lives in order to pursue their purpose, passions, and dreams, and their boldness to challenge the status quo and choose the road less traveled has made all the difference, for themselves and the world. They have taught me the meaning of grit, touched me deeply beyond words, and inspired me to live my life's purpose each and every day.

—Mao Shing Ni

This book is dedicated to my sister Grace, who lived strong. Your courage is remembered, and you are loved every day. To my parents, for your continual support and love throughout my life. And to my nephew Dylan, your intellectual spirit is infinite, just like your mother's.

—Frances Lam

Published by
Tao of Wellness Press
An Imprint of SevenStar Communications
13315 W Washington Blvd., Suite 200
Los Angeles, CA 90066
www. taoofwellness.com

© 2019 by Mao Shing Ni and Frances Lam. All rights reserved. Printed in the United States of America. No part of this book may be used or reproduced in any manner whatsoever without written permission, except in the case of brief quotations in articles or reviews.

ISBN 978-1-887575-57-7

Editing, page layout and design by Jordan Pomazon
Cover design by Justina Krakowski

A note to readers:
This book is intended to be informational and should not be considered a substitute for advice from a medical professional, whom the reader should consult before beginning any diet or exercise regiment, and before taking any dietary supplements or other medications. The author and publisher expressly disclaim responsibility for any adverse effects arising from the use or application of the information contained in this book.

TABLE OF CONTENTS

Introduction

Just about everyone knows or has lost someone dear to them to cancer. But first, let's mention some good news. Death from cancer dropped 27% over the last 25 years in the US, resulting in an estimated 2.6 million fewer cancer deaths during that period, according to the American Cancer Society. This is attributed mainly to the efforts to reduce smoking, as well as advances in detection and treatment of cancer at earlier stages.

Despite the decline in cancer death rates, 1,735,350 new cases of cancer will be diagnosed, and 609,640 people will die from the disease in 2019. A sobering fact. Recent studies in the United Kingdom concluded that one in two people will develop cancer in his or her lifetime.

Cancer is the second most common cause of death in the US, exceeded only by heart disease, and accounts for nearly one of every four deaths. Around the world, cancer claimed one out of every six deaths, or about 8.9 million people in 2016. It is estimated that there will be 23.6 million new cases of cancer each year by 2030.

Cancer has confounded modern medicine for a good part of a century. There are multiple reasons theorized by researchers as to why people develop cancer. However, according to large demographic and scientific studies, the aging process appears to be the main cause of cellular mutation that leads to the development of cancerous lesions.

Age is the biggest single risk factor for cancer. Studies show that cancer risk increases significantly after age 50, and half of all cancers occur at age 66 and above. Pause for a moment and think about that fact. In other words, when you live into your sixth decade and beyond you are more likely to develop or die of cancer than in all your prior years.

Why is aging such a threat to you getting cancer? It's pretty simple. The longer you live, the more errors your genes accumulate from infections and environmental carcinogens. As well, your cancer-fighting immunity and frequent stress response declines. Over time, these mutations are duplicated over and over as your cells divide. It's easy to see how it can eventually lead to cancer.

The facts, according to researchers, is that everyone harbors cells that may become cancerous if they are not destroyed or kept in check by your immune system. One reason that cancer is a disease of old age is that the decline of your immunity, particularly the function of thymus. The thymus is a gland that trains and produces the body's Natural Killer (NK) Cells, and it become less able to recognize and destroy cancer cells as you get older.

There are exceptions to this rule. For instance, when children or young people develop cancer. The rapid cellular division fueled by growth factors during growing years amplifies the gene errors from inherited genetic mutations or damage caused by environmental factors such as toxins and infections. This overwhelms the young immune system meant to keep cancer cells at bay. Common cancers in the young include leukemia, lymphoma, brain/spinal cord tumors, sarcoma, and reproductive cancers such as testicular in men and ovarian/breast in women.

Cancer is a ticking time bomb and it's not whether or not you will get it but a matter of "when" you will get it as you age. Sounds depressing doesn't it? After having interviewed hundreds of centenarians and deep dives into the latest research on longevity, the good news is that getting older is inevitable, but aging is not!

If you desire to prevent cancer in your lifetime or perhaps you are currently battling cancer, you must start working on your anti-aging program today. (We recommend that you read Dr. Mao's book, Secrets of Longevity to learn what centenarians do to maintain youthful function and vitality through diet, lifestyle, and mindset changes.) In the meantime, read on as this book is full of evidence-based information that will help you and your loved ones begin the journey towards health and longevity.

In this book, we have attempted to provide an overview in a user-friendly format: the critical information on the mechanism behind cancer, the diagnostic and the successful collaboration between Western and Chinese medicine. The doctors at the Tao of Wellness has worked with oncologists and cancer patients every day for more than 30 years. We have cared for many cancer patients using acupuncture and traditional Chinese medicine, nutrition, and qi gong. Alongside our oncologist colleagues whom deploy surgery, chemotherapy, radiation, and now increasingly immunotherapy with improved outcomes and quality of life.

We share the evidence-based protocols of these collaborations as well as stories of some of our patients in the hopes that you, your loved ones, or someone you know will benefit from our clinical experiences. More importantly, we want to share well researched information on prevention with as many people as possible so that you and your loved ones can avoid getting cancer in the first place.

May You Live Long and Live Strong!

Dr. Mao Shing Ni and Frances Lam, L.Ac

Chapter 1:
Why Does Cancer Happen?

My cancer scare changed my life. I'm grateful for every new,
healthy day I have. It has helped me prioritize my life.
— *Olivia Newton-John*

You are made up of trillions of cells. Normally, your cells divide and multiply on a precise schedule, so that your body has the correct amount and type of cells. This allows the body to maintain, repair, and restore tissues and functions.

Cancer happens when one or more abnormal cells begin to divide uncontrollably, and form masses of tissue called tumors. Tumors can be benign or malignant. Benign tumors do not spread and are harmless. A lipoma is an example of a benign tumor that's composed of fat cells that are mostly harmless. A tumor is called malignant when it shows signs that it has spread throughout the body from the point of origin. When it starts to spread beyond the original site, it has metastasized.

Cancer cells invade the body through the lymph system and blood flow. They do this by dividing, growing, and making new blood vessels to feed on, this process is called angiogenesis. In contrast to tumors, blood cancers like leukemia start from blood cells and do not form solid tumors. Instead, the cancer cells build in the blood and sometimes in the bone marrow. The symptoms often show up as fever, night sweats, fatigue, joint pain, swollen lymph nodes, and weight loss.

What makes normal cells turn rogue and grow abnormally? That's the question cancer researchers and doctors have been trying to answer. Fortunately, we now know more than ever about the mechanism of cancer. For example, we know that cancers begin with gene mutation, meaning the cells' DNA has changed or been damaged causing it to no longer act normally. Gene mutations can be inherited or caused by environmental factors such as carcinogens, infections, and obesity. Yes, you read that right— obesity! Being overweight profoundly increases the risk of cancer, especially ones that are hormonally sensitive like breast, ovarian, prostate, and many others. Primarily though, aging is the biggest cause of cancer. That's why most obituaries for the elderly list cancer as the cause of death.

To find cures for this devastating disease we must understand "why does cancer happen?" In this chapter, we share research ranging from ancient to modern times that has helped in the progress of prevention and treatment of cancer.

Cancer Is an Aging Problem

Age is the biggest single risk factor for cancer. The risk of cancer increases significantly after age 50, and half of all cancers occur at age 66 and above. According to the National Cancer Institute, one-quarter of new cancer diagnoses are in people aged 65 to 74. The longer we live, the more errors our genes accumulate. Over time, these mutations can lead to cancer.

How then do we know how well we are aging? Telomeres, the ends of DNA strands, can serve as molecular markers of aging. Their deterioration has been linked to the change of normal cells into cancer cells. Getting older is inevitable, aging is not—so start working on your anti-aging program today.

(We recommend that you read Dr. Mao's book Secrets of Longevity to learn what centenarians do to maintain youthfulness through diet, lifestyle, and mindset changes.)

Do You have Oncogenes?

Oncogenes are genes that have mutated and have the potential to cause the growth of cancer cells. Mutations can be inherited or due to exposure to substances in the environment that cause cancer. For example, researchers have found that 5 to 10 percent of all cancers are influenced by inherited genetic mutations.

There are more than 50 specific hereditary cancers which a person may be predisposed to developing. And genetic tests can reveal if a person has inherited the mutation. However, even if you inherit a genetic mutation, other factors can influence how the mutation will develop.

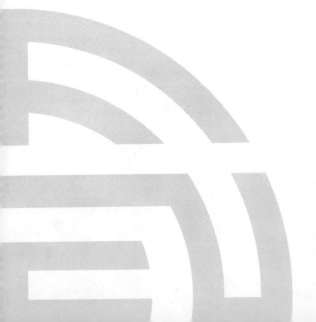

P53—Proofreading Genes that Protect the Body Against Insurrection

P53 is a gene found in all cells, except red blood cells. Sometimes called guardians of the genome or the proofreader gene, p53 reads all your other genes for errors. It protects the body by rooting out cells that have become abnormal or malignant. P53 works in a three-step process: arrest, repair, and apoptosis.

- Arrest stops the cell from replicating suspicious DNA.
- Repair attempts to fix damaged DNA so the cell can continue working.
- Apoptosis destroys the cell in order to stop it from spreading abnormal DNA.

This is how your immune system keeps bad cells from growing into cancers. Unfortunately, p53 is mutated or broken by about 40% of all cancers. And the remaining cancers frequently find other ways to suppress its functions.

It's not all bad news though. Researchers have found a way to turn the p53 proofreader genes back on in rats with widespread metastatic cancer. When they did the cancer was subdued. Time will tell, but this could be good news for humans.

A Weakened Thymus Makes You Susceptible to Cancer

Everyone harbors cells that may become cancerous if they are not destroyed or kept in check by our immune system. That is why it's so important to have a strong immune system, so that it can destroy suspicious cells. However, when the immune system becomes overwhelmed or loses its ability to recognize a rogue cell, they escape and multiply.

One reason that cancer is a disease of old age is that the immune system is less able to combat cancer as you get older. This is because as you age your thymus is less able to train and produce natural killer (NK) cells. These cells are responsible for fighting both tumors and infected cells. As a result, your body has trouble recognizing and destroying cancer cells.

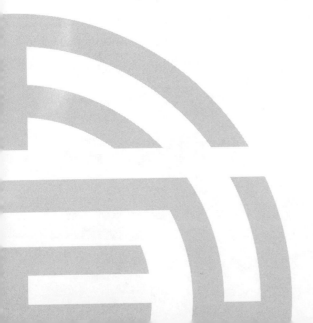

Chronic Inflammation Is the Root of Many Evils

Chronic inflammation causes trauma to the body that the immune system attempts to fix by generating free radicals. These free radicals spread throughout the body and blood in order to clean up the damage.

But if the body becomes overwhelmed by this trauma, the response to fix it can go on too long. Too many free radicals can cause oxidative damage to tissue. Oxidative damage is when your body's free radicals and antioxidants are out of balance, leading to functional breakdown and cell damage. If left unchecked by your immune system, it can go on to make cancer cells.

Chronic inflammation stems from many factors, such as:
- Poor diet
- Exposure to toxins
- Sedentary lifestyle
- Stress
- Injuries

Oxygen Deprivation Drives Cancer Growth

Cancer appears to feed off oxygen deprivation, or hypoxia as it's clinically known. Studies show that intermittent hypoxia can increase the risk of developing cancer, as well as causing mutated cells to spread beyond their incubation site. When hypoxia occurs, the body throws off free radicals and increases tissue inflammation. During this, cancer cells actively seek oxygen and energy by forming new blood vessels and invading surrounding tissues. Researchers have found that intermittent hypoxia is one of the causes of metastasis in triple negative breast cancer.

One example of hypoxia is sleep apnea. Sleep apnea occurs when breathing is periodically interrupted during sleep, usually by a blockage in the airway. If you wake up tired, even after an adequate amount of sleep, ask your doctor to test you for sleep apnea.

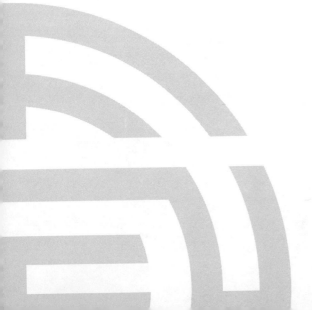

Watch Out for Environmental Damage to Your DNA

There are several environmental carcinogens that damage our DNA:

- Chemicals
- Smoke
- Radiation
- Pesticides
- Smog
- Diet-related agents
- Infections

External and internal factors affect everyone differently, but they all carry the risk of causing changes to our cells and potentially leading to cancerous lesions. For instance, studies showed that simply being exposed to smog increased the risk of breast cancer in women. Additionally, world-wide investigations have revealed that a commonly used herbicide, glyphosate, has been linked to increased Non-Hodgkin's lymphoma and potentially other cancers. This is just to mention a few environmental factors.

Obesity and Excess Weight Lead to Cancer

In 2016, an estimated 1.97 billion adults and over 338 million children were overweight or obese around the world. There is strong evidence that being overweight or obese is a cause of numerous cancers, for example:

- Esophagus (adenocarcinoma)
- Mouth
- Pharynx and larynx
- Stomach
- Pancreas
- Liver
- Gallbladder
- Colorectal
- Breast (postmenopausal)
- Ovarian
- Endometrium
- Prostate
- Kidney

Besides cancer, obesity also increases the risk of heart disease and diabetes.

Eating Lunch Meat Increases
Colorectal Cancer Risk

Harvard University researchers reviewed 30 studies of colorectal cancer and found that eating around 50 grams (almost 2 ounces) of processed meat a day is associated with about a 20% increase in colorectal cancer. Colorectal cancer targets the large intestine (colon) and is the third most diagnosed cancer in men. Studies also show a similarly increased risk with daily red meat (beef, pork, lamb) consumption.

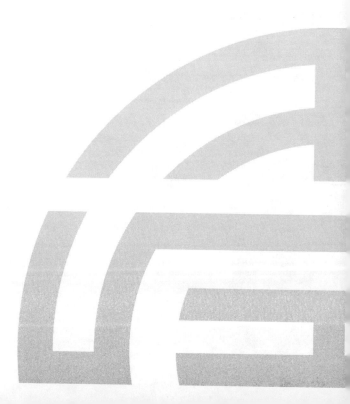

High GI Is Bad for Joe's Prostate

Glycemic index (GI) measures how quickly foods cause increases in blood glucose levels. A study of 3,100 subjects found that consuming foods with a high GI was associated with an 88% greater risk for prostate cancer. High GI foods are 70 or higher on the 100-point GI scale, and consist of refined, processed, white foods. Examples are:

- White bread
- White potato
- White rice
- Processed cereal
- Pizza
- Fruit juices
- Sugar-sweetened soft drinks

In general, beans and legumes have a lower GI score.

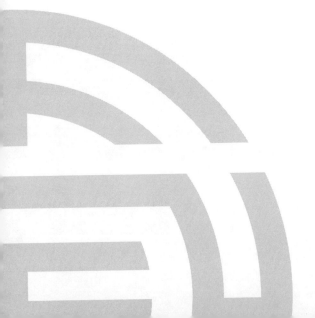

Rethinking Barbecuing, Grilling, and Frying Meat

Heterocyclic amines (HCAs) are chemicals formed when meat is cooked using high-temperature methods. These methods include pan-frying, grilling directly over an open flame, or smoking. Studies have shown that a high intake of HCA meat may be associated with the risk of such cancers as:

- Colorectal
- Breast
- Prostate
- Pancreas
- Lung
- Stomach
- Esophagus

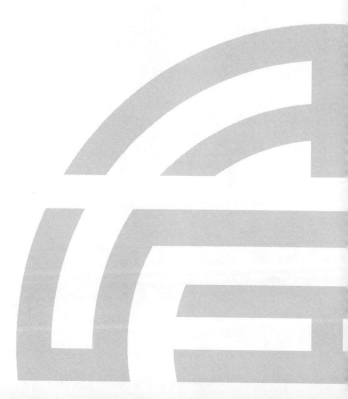

Hungry Cancer Cells Feed on Sugar

All cells, whether healthy or cancerous, need energy to function. In particular cancer cells, which multiply quickly and have a constant need for fuel. Their fuel often comes from sugar. A number of studies have shown a strong correlation between high sucrose sugar intake and high insulin levels. This results in increased risks of cancers like:

- Pancreatic
- Colon
- Breast

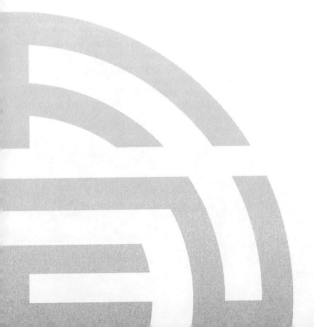

Diabetes Increases Risk Factor for Cancer

An Australian study has shown that people with type 1 or type 2 diabetes are more often diagnosed with certain types of cancer. They are also more likely to die from cancer than people without diabetes. The highest risks the researchers saw were for cancers that affect the:

- Pancreas
- Liver
- Endometrium
- Kidneys
- Thyroid
- Gallbladder
- Blood cells
- Bone marrow

If you have diabetes, it's highly recommended you get screened for cancer.

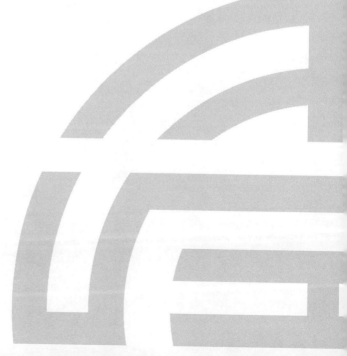

Be Careful Where You Decide to Move

The evidence between diet and cancer is backed up even more when you look at the variation of specific cancers around the world and the occurrence of cancer shifting. Cancer shifting describes the phenomenon of cancer statistics for a specific race and how it changes when relocated to another country or region. For example, Asians that move to the West have a higher rate of both breast and prostate cancer than their counterparts in their home countries. According to one study, that translates to at least a 25 times higher rate of prostate and 10 times higher rate of breast cancer after moving to the West. Furthermore, the incidence of prostate cancer is highest in Scandinavian countries at 22 cases per 100,000 people and lowest in Asia at 5 per 100,000. The US rate is 9 cases per 100,000. However, Asian men who immigrated to the US developed similar prostate cancer rates as US men, strongly linking environmental factors to cancer.

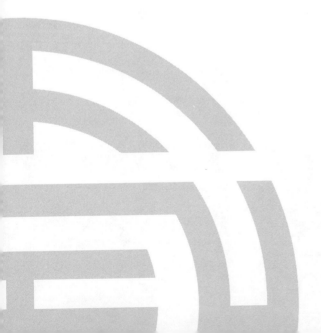

Heavy Metals are Carcinogenic and Teratogenic

Exposure to heavy metals can be found everywhere, in the food we eat, the air we breathe, and in the water we drink. Many studies have confirmed the cancer causing properties of industrial heavy metals such as mercury, arsenic, and cadmium. Some studies have found that besides causing cancer, heavy metals are also teratogenic. This means they can cause genetic defects and mutations to offspring several generations beyond the person originally exposed.

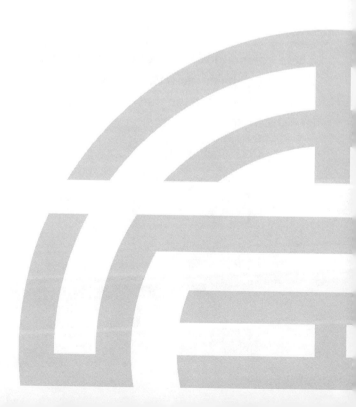

Toxins, Toxins Everywhere

The International Agency for Research on Cancer has identified 415 known or suspected carcinogens in our bodies. Researchers at both the University of California Davis and Los Angeles conducted studies where they measured food-borne toxin exposure in children and adults. This was done by pinpointing foods with high levels of toxic compounds and determining how much of these foods were consumed. According to the researchers' findings, the family members in the study were at a high risk of exposure to:

- Arsenic
- Dieldrin
- DDE
- Dioxins
- Acrylamide
- Pesticides

These compounds have been linked to cancer, developmental disabilities, birth defects, and other conditions. Preschool children involved in the study were at a particularly high risk.

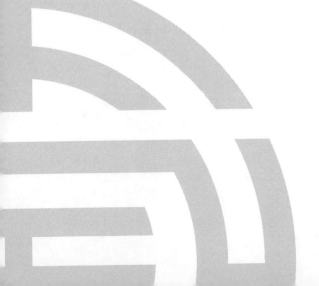

Everyday Chemicals, Some Obvious and Others Not so Obvious

Everyday chemicals present in our environment have been linked to cancer. These include:

- Cosmetics
- Paint
- Air fresheners
- Pesticides
- Lead
- Wood dust
- Car fumes
- Cigarette smoke
- Radon
- Flame retardants
- Formaldehyde
- Dust
- Mold
- Fungus
- Fuel emissions (from cars, landscaping equipment, leaf blowers, etc.)

Research has shown that we can reduce cancer rates by limiting our exposure to toxins.

Off-Gas Damage to Protective Proteins in Genes

Studies have shown that chemicals that are off-gassed from formaldehyde glue and flame retardants damage proteins in our body. These same proteins would normally restore and preserve the chromosome structure of other proteins. For example, the BRCA gene is a tumor suppressor gene that helps to prevent breast cancer by repairing damaged DNA. But in some people suppressor genes do not function properly and the gene is altered by toxic chemicals in a way that leads to cancer.

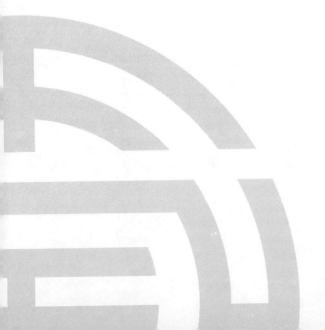

A Radioactive Off-Gas

Radon is a radioactive gas that comes from the natural disintegration of uranium in soil and rock. Large tracts of homes around the world were built on soil that off-gasses radon. This has caused radon to become the number one cause of lung cancer among non-smokers, according to the US Environmental Protection Agency (EPA). Overall, radon is the second leading cause of lung cancer and responsible for 21,000 lung cancer deaths every year. According to the World Health Organization (WHO), radon causes up to 15% of lung cancers worldwide. The levels of radon inside your house can be measured by hiring a radon inspector.

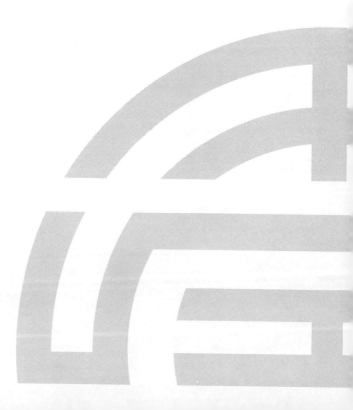

Chemotherapy and Radiation May Lead to Future Cancer

Chemotherapy and radiation are the standard treatment protocols for cancer. The downside is that secondary cancers can emerge months or years after as a result of the treatment for the initial cancer. According to a study published in the Journal of the National Cancer Institute, certain chemotherapeutic drugs raise the risk of secondary cancers, particularly acute myeloid leukemia (AML), by up to five times. This is because chemotherapy agents are highly toxic. Their goal is to eradicate the cancer or tumor, but by doing so the chemical also annihilates the good cells too.

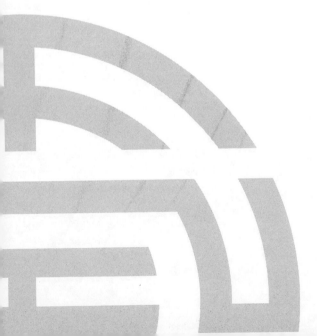

Some Drugs Have Been Linked to Cancer But Are Still Prescribed

Some drugs need further safety studies. Actos (pioglitazone), an oral diabetes medication made by the company Takeda, is one such example. The FDA held two three-year studies on the drug to measure its effects. The results showed a higher incidence of bladder cancer in patients who took Actos versus those who took other drugs. As a result of these studies, the FDA required that Takeda undertake a 10-year study of the drug's link to bladder cancer. Despite lawsuits and FDA review, Actos is still prescribed in the US even though the drug has been pulled from the market in Germany, France, and India.

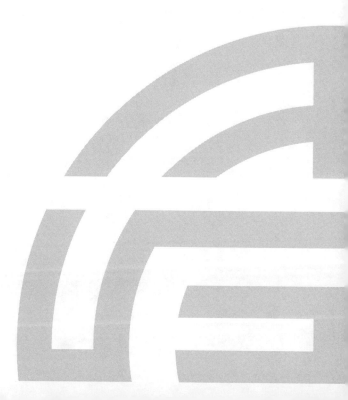

Watch out for Drugs That Suppress Your Immune System

Many people who suffer from autoimmune diseases, as well as those who receive organ transplants, take medications to suppress the immune system. This is so the inflammatory process can be stopped, or in the case of transplants, the body won't reject the organ. The downside of these drugs is that they make the immune system less able to detect and destroy cancer cells or fight off infections that cause cancer.

Research has shown that people who use immunosuppressant drugs are at a higher risk of a large number of different cancers. The most common cancers that occur in these individuals are non-Hodgkin lymphoma (NHL) and lung, kidney, and liver cancers. Some of these cancers can also be caused by infections like the Epstein-Barr virus (EBV), and hepatitis B and C.

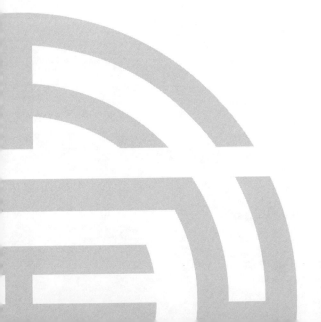

Hormone Replacement Therapy (HRT) Has a High Price

As we age, our hormones decline. In an attempt to replenish them, people turn to hormone replacement therapy (HRT). As a result, they sacrifice their health, increasing the odds of cancer.

By the mid 1970's, HRT was linked to endometrial and breast cancer for women. Further studies in the 1990's verified the link to cancer, causing the National Institute of Health to begin their own study on the safety of estrogen. Furthermore, a discovery was made during the Women's Health Initiative, a large study involving 25,000 women using both estrogen and progestin. The discovery linked the use of estrogen and progestin to increased breast cancer risk and stroke. This prompted an abrupt termination of the study. Other studies also show links to colon and ovarian cancer.

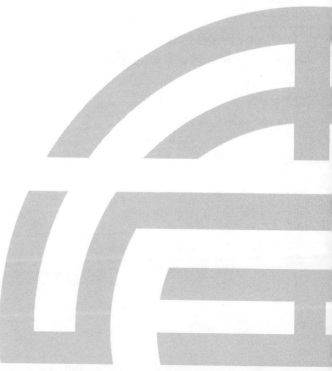

Do Cell Phones and Radiofrequency Cause Cancer?

Every day we are exposed to non-ionizing radiation. It comes in the form of:

- Visible light
- Radio frequency (RF)
- Microwave ovens
- Televisions
- Cell phones

It was long thought that non-ionizing radiation had enough energy to excite atoms, but not enough energy to change the structure of the molecule. That might not be the case anymore. A combined analysis of two case-control studies conducted in Sweden reported statistically significant trends. The study showed an increased risk of brain cancer for people who began using cell phones before the age of 20. The International Agency for Research on Cancer, an arm of WHO, classified cell phone use as "possibly carcinogenic to humans," based on limited evidence from human studies. Until there's definitive clarity, it is best to use corded headsets and the speakerphone when using cell phones.

Should You Be Concerned About the X-Ray Security Scanner at the Airport?

X-rays, CT scans, and nuclear imaging use ionizing radiation. When atoms are ionized the cell either dies or repairs itself. If the cell cannot repair itself it mutates, leading to DNA damage that can increase your chances of cancer.

Airport body scanners uses low level X-rays that are about 0.25 microsievert per encounter. For frequent flyers, experts recommend a safety limit of 250 microsieverts per year. In other words, that would be 1,000 scans per year, if the scanner is operating at its highest power.

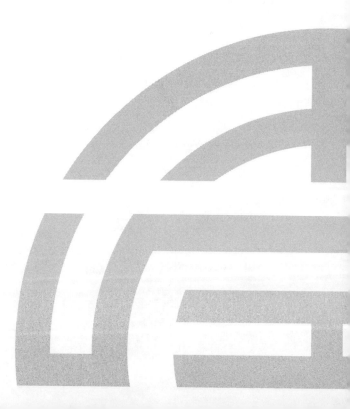

Infections Cause One in Seven Cancer Cases

Infections by certain viruses, bacteria, and parasites are one of the biggest and most preventable causes of cancer worldwide. According to worldwide studies, 2.2 million of the total 14 million new cancer cases in 2012 were caused by infections. That's about one in every seven cases. Viruses and bacteria can do this by embedding their own genes into healthy cells, causing long-term inflammation. The constant inflammation can lead to cancer by triggering free radicals that stimulate mutations in the cells. Changes to healthy cells can also affect the immune system, weakening your defenses. Infections that can cause this include:

- Helicobacter pylori
- Human papillomavirus
- Hepatitis B & C
- Epstein-Barr virus

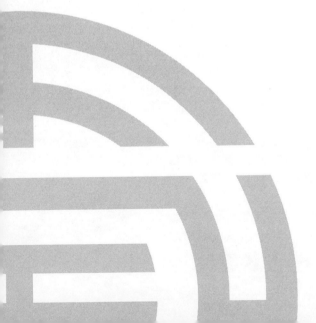

Acute and Chronic Stress Can Stimulate Cancer Progression

Acute or short term stress that lasts for a few minutes, hours, or a day or two activates the brain's fight-or-flight response. This is the body's natural survival mechanism, and as such it's perfectly normal. On the other hand, chronic stress, which can affect us for weeks, months, or even years, is not. Chronic stress can provoke a flood of hormones from the adrenal glands such as cortisol and adrenaline. High, constant cortisol levels can affect other functions of the body such as the digestive, reproductive, and immune systems, as well as our emotions and development.

Studies have shown how both acute and chronic stress can stimulate cancer progression. It does this by weakening the immune system and encouraging new tumor-feeding blood vessels to form. According to a study published in the Journal of Cancer Prevention, "stress hormones can have a significant impact on protecting cancer cells from undergoing anoikis—a type of programmed cell death, thus providing an advantage for metastasis to occur."

Xenoestrogen Is a Good Reason to Eat Only Organic

Many chemicals cause estrogenic-like responses from your body. These estrogen-stimulating chemicals are collectively called xenoestrogen. Examples of xenoestrogen are:

- Pesticides
- Polychlorinated biphenyls (PCB's)
- Formaldehyde

When estrogen is abnormally high in a woman's body she may develop a condition called estrogen dominance. This can result in:

- Menstrual irregularity
- Weight gain
- Premenstrual syndrome (PMS)
- Polycystic ovarian syndrome (PCOS)
- Endometriosis
- Fibroids
- Cysts

Studies have also linked xenoestrogens to increased risks of cancers of the:

- Breast
- Ovaries
- Uterus
- Pancreas

Chapter 2:
How Cancer Can Be Prevented

Maintaining order rather than correcting disorder is the ultimate principle of healing. To cure disease after it has appeared is like digging a well after one feels thirsty or forging weapons after the war has already begun.
— *Yellow Emperor's Classic of Medicine*

Since 1971, the overall incidence of cancer has risen by 24%. In 2000, there were 1.2 million new cases of cancer in the US alone. In 2018, new cases of cancer have been estimated to have risen to 1.7 million. In particular, incidences of breast, prostate, thyroid, and lymph gland cancers have all risen sharply. Today, close to 40% of men and women will develop cancer in their lifetimes. Even taking into account the US population growth over the last 40 years, that percentage is far too high.

While death from cancer has dropped 27% in the last 25 years due to improved screening and early intervention, it's clear from the sharp rise in cancer rates that not enough is being done. Especially considering many cases are due to environmental factors that are preventable. The US cancer establishment conducts minimal research on exposure to a wide range of avoidable industrial carcinogens in the air, water, soil, workplace, and in consumer products such as carcinogenic prescription drugs and diagnostic medical radiation.

Just as critically, the cancer establishment has failed to do its part. The public, media, Congress, and regulatory agencies have not been properly educated and warned of avoidable carcinogens. This failure to warn the public of cancer risks is in striking contrast to the cancer establishment's stream of releases claiming the latest advances in screening, treatment, and basic research.

The highest priority for research and prevention funding has been directed towards "secondary" prevention. While important, this only focuses on screening, early detection, and chemoprevention through drug use. Minimal research is being done on "primary" prevention for avoidable causes of cancer, such as environmental carcinogens. Primary prevention is essential for reducing cancer incidence around the world.

The persistent carelessness of governmental and health agencies towards cancer prevention is reflected in the EPA's position on glyphosate. Glyphosate is the herbicide ingredient in weed killer, and the EPA states it is "not likely to cause cancer." This is in direct contradiction to research by the World Health Organization and California's Office of Environmental Health Hazard that "glyphosate is known to cause cancer!"

Thousands of new chemicals continue to be unleashed on the environment each and every year. Even after spending over 40 years and an estimated $200 billion there has been a negligible amount of money spent on cancer prevention research, education, and enforcement. The two exceptions to this have been informing people of the dangers of smoking and alcohol. But after so much time and money, one would expect more to have been done.

This lack of commitment to the primary prevention of avoidable causes of cancer is a travesty that has resulted in an immeasurable amount of unneeded suffering, loss of human life, and financial ruin.

Understanding how and why cancer happens can help people avoid this truly unnecessary disease. Each person needs to learn how to avoid anything that causes their normally healthy functions to decline or become abnormal. It's also important to understand what creates mutations to cells' DNA. The concept is simple but requires constant learning, the will to change, and the creation of an environment that allows for the changes to be lasting. There are, however, certain things we cannot change, such as our genetics. Although research is underway on genetic testing and gene editing tools to possibly repair defective or mutated genes, no reliable method has been found.

Until there are proven methods to safely edit genes, research has shown other tried and true ways to deal with even genetically predisposed cancer. In this chapter you'll learn how application of epigenetics can help do exactly that. You'll learn that some foods can be helpful, while others are harmful. We will also discuss simple ways for you to detoxify and clear your body of the buildup of carcinogens over many years. You'll also discover evidence-based ways to improve your body's functions and slow down, and even reverse, the aging process—as aging is the biggest carcinogen of them all.

Keep Your BMI and WHR Within Optimum Range

One of our cancer prevention recommendations is to keep your weight within the healthy range and avoid weight gain in adult life. Studies show strong evidence that obesity is a cause of numerous cancers, like:

- Pancreatic
- Liver
- Esophagus
- Colon
- Kidney
- Endometrium
- Breast

High Body Mass Index (BMI) and waist and hip ratio (WHR) are also a probable cause of cancers of the:

- Mouth
- Pharynx
- Larynx
- Stomach
- Gallbladder
- Ovary
- Prostate

There are many online calculators to determine your BMI. To calculate your WHR simply divide your waist circumference by your hip circumference. Maintaining a healthy weight throughout your life is one of the most important ways for you to protect against cancer. Medically, being overweight or obese means your BMI exceeds 25 and your WHR is higher than 1.

Keep your cancer risks, not to mention also heart disease and diabetes risks, low by keeping your weight within the healthy range.

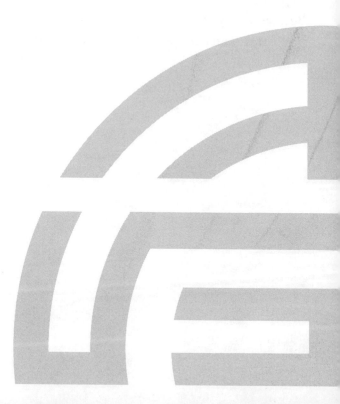

Reduce Your Screen Time

Sedentary lifestyles and lack of physical activity are globally widespread issues. According to a new study, American adults spend more than 11 hours per day watching and interacting with screens. That's up from nine hours, 32 minutes just four years ago. Screen time is a marker of sedentary living and is a cause of weight gain in children and adults. In addition, people watching screens are often exposed to marketing of unhealthy foods and drinks, and may be consuming energy-dense snacks and drinks while watching. All of these can contribute to weight gain.

There is strong evidence that physical activity protects against colon, breast, and endometrial cancer, as well as helping prevent excess weight gain. One of the most important cancer prevention steps you can take is to be physically active as part of everyday life. Besides saving yourself from cancer down the road, you are also protecting yourself against heart disease, stroke, and diabetes.

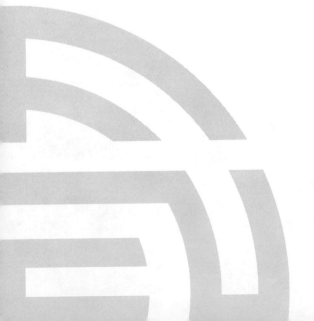

Maternal Programming to Prevent Obesity in Children

Most women are not aware of the impact of their behavior and health on the well-being of their unborn children. Chinese medicine has long advocated healthy maternal programming. As documented in the Yellow Emperor's Classic of Medicine, "the food an expectant mother consumed, the thoughts and emotions that she experienced and the activities that she engaged in during her entire pregnancy shall have a direct impact on her unborn children's health."

Studies now show that the environment of the womb plays an important role in disease risk and traits developed later in life. Factors such as nutrition or infection influence the fetus and can cause risk of weight gain and obesity both in childhood and adulthood. Infants of mothers who are obese tend to have greater fetal size and increased fat mass, both are risk factors for obesity and by extension cancer. So the message is simple: eat well during pregnancy, avoid gaining more than 35 pounds, and avoid stress and tension. Your baby will thank you.

Your Microbiome Is Your Best Defense

There is growing evidence that the bacteria residing in the colon, otherwise known as the microbiome, may hold the key to cancer prevention. A study published in Science Translational Medicine showed how dysbiosis (an imbalance of the microbiome) can lead to cancer formation. The researchers discovered that intestinal dysbiosis can trigger an inflammatory response in the intestinal tract that can lead to diseases such as Crohn's or cancer of colorectal, breast, and liver.

The intestinal microbiome helps protect the intestinal lining. It also serves as a gatekeeper that allows nutrients to be absorbed into the bloodstream while blocking disease-causing toxins from passing through. When it fails, it can lead to the breakdown of the immune system. Worse, it can subject tissues and cells to damage, ultimately resulting in mutations that may lead to cancer. Furthermore, the microbiome has also been shown to be involved with the development of overweight and obesity.

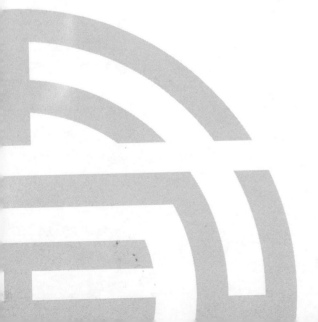

Restoring your microbiome to a healthy state is simple but diligent work. It requires that you stop eating processed and sugary foods, avoid antibiotics unless it's absolutely necessary, and increase your consumption of probiotic-rich foods such as:

- Kefir
- Kimchee
- Kombucha
- Sauerkraut
- Miso
- Yogurt

You should also take a probiotic supplement from a reputable company.

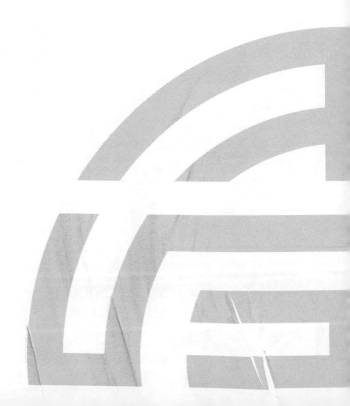

Breastfeeding is Good for Both Mother and Baby

There is definitive evidence that breastfeeding is good for both mother and child. For mothers, it protects against breast cancer, and it has also been found to lower the risk of type 2 diabetes. For infants it helps protect against obesity and the cancers that are influenced by it. Excess body fat tends to persist into adulthood and can increase the risk of cancer, asthma, and type 2 diabetes. Other health benefits of breastfeeding include protection against infections in infancy and immune system development. So breastfeed away to keep cancer away.

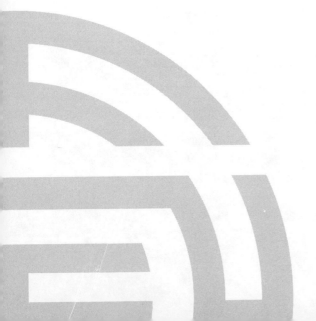

To Drink or Not to Drink, That Is the Question

Experts from around the world have concluded that for cancer prevention it's best not to drink alcohol. It has been determined that consumption of alcoholic drinks is a cause for cancers of the:

- Mouth
- Pharynx
- Larynx
- Esophagus
- Liver
- Colorectal
- Breast
- Stomach

Unfortunately, there is no bottom threshold of alcohol consumption which does not increase cancer risk, at least for some cancers. Sounds depressing, doesn't it?

Why is alcohol bad? Your body metabolizes the ethanol in alcoholic drinks into acetaldehyde, a compound not found in your body otherwise. Acetaldehyde can damage cellular DNA and generate free radicals that damage more DNA. Alcohol also impairs your body's ability to break down and absorb nutrients such as vitamins A, folate, C, D, E, and carotenoids. It also increases the blood levels in estrogen, which is linked to the risk of breast cancer. The important factor is the amount of ethanol consumed regardless of the type. Whether it's beer, wine, spirits, or any other alcoholic drink, they all have a similar impact on cancer risk. If you must consume alcoholic drinks, drink little and infrequently.

Choose a Plant Based Diet and You'll be Better Off

The "Western" diet is full of foods which have been shown in studies to elevate cancer, heart disease, and diabetes risks. The diet often contains:

- Sugar
- Salt
- Fats
- Red meat
- Refined food
- Processed food
- Fast food

According to Louise Meincke of the World Cancer Research Fund, "the increasing availability, affordability and acceptability of fast foods is contributing to rising rates of obesity worldwide." Sugar and refined, starchy foods have a high glycemic index. This means they spike insulin and insulin growth factor (IGF-1), thus raising the risk of cancer. Likewise, fast foods and processed foods have additives and byproducts that may be carcinogenic. Additionally, fats, salts, and red meat all collectively contribute to the disease process. This is especially true of conventionally raised animals with hormones, antibiotics, and corn-feed.

Large demographic studies around the world have concluded that plant based diet like those associated with Chinese and Mediterranean diets is healthiest. It lowers the risk of modern diseases, such as cancer, heart disease, and diabetes. Dietary patterns that are linked to a lower risk of cancer consistently feature high consumption of:

- Whole grains
- Vegetables
- Fruits
- Nuts
- Seeds
- Beans
- Legumes

Be sure to get at least 30 grams of fiber and 5 servings of vegetables and fruits in your diet daily. If you must eat animal products, limit your weekly consumption to 12-18 oz. of free range, organic, grass-fed meat or wild caught seafood.

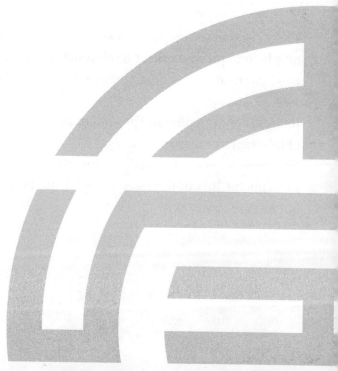

Mother Knows Best—Eat Your Broccoli

Not all vegetables are made equal. There exists a number of superfoods chock-full of special nutrients that can help you prevent cancer from forming in the first place. Topping the list of superfoods are cruciferous vegetables known for their cancer fighting properties. Cruciferous veggies include:

- Broccoli
- Cauliflower
- Brussels sprouts
- Cabbage
- Kale
- Wasabi
- Horseradish
- Mustard
- Radish
- Watercress

These contain sulforaphane, a sulfur-containing compound that may help to prevent cancer by eliminating potential carcinogens and by activating tumor suppressor genes in cells.

Interestingly, cruciferous sprouts contain ten times higher levels of sulforaphane than mature vegetables. Boiling and microwaving has been shown to reduce sulforaphanes, whereas steaming prevents the loss of the essential nutrient. So eat your broccoli, but be sure to steam it.

Don't Like Broccoli?
You May Find DIM More Palatable

For many years, researchers at the University of Minnesota have been studying compounds that may prevent cancer. Their groundbreaking research has uncovered the cancer prevention properties of many dietary compounds, including indole-3-carbinol (I3C) and diindolylmethane (DIM).

I3C is formed from a substance called glucobrassicin, which is found in such vegetables as:

- Broccoli
- Brussels sprouts
- Cabbage
- Collards
- Cauliflower
- Kale
- Mustard greens
- Turnips
- Rutabagas

I3C is formed when these vegetables are cut, chewed, or cooked. On the other hand, DIM is a natural substance generated when the body breaks down I3C.

I3C and DIM have been found to adjust the activity of enzymes to the body's needs. One example is aromatase, which is involved in the metabolism and elimination of many compounds in the body, such as steroid hormones, drugs, carcinogens, and toxins.

DIM is a natural aromatase inhibitor that helps support fat loss and healthy estrogen metabolism. Its other health benefits include anti-inflammatory and anticancer effects. It was also shown to increase bone mass, which may have implications for patients with osteoporosis. DIM is available in supplement form.

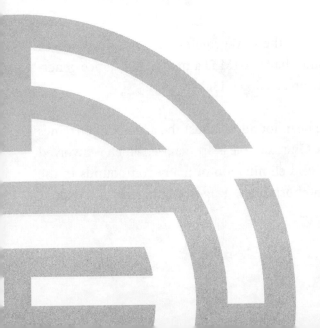

Find Sweetness in Your Life, Not Your Sugar Intake

The average American consumes nearly 240 pounds of sugar per year. Most of that excess sugar is stored as fat in your body, this elevates cancer risk and can suppress your immune functions. When study subjects were given sugar, their white blood cell count decreased significantly for several hours afterwards. This is true for a variety of sugars, including:

- Fructose
- Glucose
- Honey
- Orange juice

Instead of sugary drinks, opt for water or unsweetened drinks, such as tea or coffee, without added sugar. Fruit juices should be avoided, instead eat the whole fruit. But you can flavor your water with fruit slices, like orange, strawberry, or cucumber. Tea and coffee are great choices which have been shown to protect against cancer. For natural sweeteners that are safe try stevia, monk fruit extract, or a small amount of coconut sugar.

Don't Stress Over Things You Can't Change

Chronic stress is damaging to your health and wellbeing. Whether it's caring for a sick loved one, dealing with unemployment, or going through a difficult divorce, long term stress can weaken your immune system. Chronic stress helps cancer grow and spread in a number of ways. It can increase the production of certain growth factors that increase your blood supply, feeding the development of tumors. And stress hormones such as cortisol can inhibit a process called anoikis—a form of programmed cell death which kills diseased cells and prevents them from spreading.

There are numerous ways and methods for lowering stress and its negative physical responses, ranging from exercise to meditation and getting a good night's sleep. However, the most critical change you can make is to shift your mindset and stop worrying about what you have no control over. In other words, live in the moment, since you cannot change what happened yesterday or control what will happen tomorrow. Let go of trying to please or change someone as you have no control over what someone's thinking or how they are behaving. You may feel relieved once you decide to stop stressing over what you can't change, and instead focus on only what you can change. Oh, and don't forget to meditate every day.

Oxygenate with Breathing Practices

Studies show that oxygen plays an important role in cancer growth. Hypoxia, or oxygen deprivation, can promote cancer cell migration and remote metastasis. When there is an insufficient amount of oxygen in the bloodstream, the body produces free radicals which increase tissue inflammation and destruction. This results in cancer cells actively seeking out oxygen and energy by forming new blood vessels and invading surrounding tissues.

The cure for hypoxia is simple: just breath! However, you may suffer from conditions that prevent healthy oxygen levels in your blood. Examples of low oxygen risk conditions include:

- Obstructive sleep apnea
- Asthma
- Emphysema
- Chronic obstructive pulmonary disorder (COPD)
- Low blood pressure
- Heart disease
- Hyperventilation
- Anemia

Besides receiving proper treatment for what's causing hypoxia, we suggest a daily practice of breathing exercises, such as qi gong and breathing meditation. Keeping your body fully oxygenated means increased energy, better health, and reduced cancer risks.

Staying Physically Active Is the Best Insurance

Many occupations involve long periods of sitting. People whose work is sedentary need to take special care to build physical activity into their everyday lives. Both adults and children should minimize the amount of time they are sedentary, especially those in front of a screen or device. Studies now equate sedentary lifestyles with having similar risk factors to your health as smoking a pack of cigarettes a day. Besides an increased cancer rate, obesity and hip and lower back pain are common complaints for those who are sedentary.

The WHO advises adults to be active daily and do at least 150 minutes of moderate physical activity, such as:
- Walking
- Cycling
- Household chores
- Gardening
- Swimming
- Dancing
- Tai chi
- Qi gong
- Yoga

The rising popularity of standing desks, cycle-desks, and treadmill desks are good options for those with jobs that require them to be stationary. Get up often to have a drink or use the restroom, leave your desk and walk to lunch even if you bring your own, and stay as active as possible for the best insurance against cancer.

Mushrooms Are Magical, Potent Cancer Fighters

Mushrooms have been found to be protective against cancer. In particular, increased mushroom consumption was significantly associated with a lower risk of breast cancer development. Other studies have found medicinal mushrooms help the immune response and anti-tumor mechanisms. These immune effects appear to happen due to the mushroom's stimulation of immune cells such as monocytes, natural killer cells, and dendritic cells.

According to the National Cancer Institute, medicinal mushrooms have been approved adjuncts to standard cancer treatments in Japan and China for more than 30 years. They have an extensive clinical history of safe use on their own, or combined with radiation therapy or chemotherapy. The most prominent medicinal, cancer fighting mushrooms include:

- Ganoderma (reishi)
- Coriolus (turkey tail)
- Lentinus (shitake)
- Grifola (maitake)
- Hericium (lion's mane)
- Agaricus
- Polyporus (umbrella polypore)
- Cordyceps
- Calvatia (puffball)
- Inonotus (Chaga)
- Poria

These are all available in supplement forms. Clinical trials in cancer patients have demonstrated that medicinal mushrooms are generally well tolerated.

Keep Your Immune System Strong and Thymus Function Healthy

Aging is due to functional decline of the human body. Functional decline in such a critical role as the immune system increases cancer risks, hence why aging is considered a major carcinogen. A key producer of the immune systems natural killer (NK) cells is the thymus gland. When you are young, your thymus gland is about the size of a walnut, and by the time you turn 60 it has atrophied to the size of a pea.

Your stock of natural killer cells is built up when you are young, and as you age the function of the thymus is diminished. It is largely degenerated and barely identifiable in elderly adults, consisting mostly of fatty tissue. Atrophy of the thymus has been linked to loss of immune function in the elderly, susceptibility to infection, and cancer.

To boost thymus function you can simply take your index and third finger and gently tap the middle of your sternum 30-50 times daily. Studies also show supplementing with bovine thymus extract, astragalus root, ligustri seed, and other Chinese herbs can help support healthy thymus function.

Chapter 3:
How Is Cancer Diagnosed?

Since I had cancer I've realized that every day is a bonus.
– Geoffrey Boycott

Receiving a cancer diagnosis is likely the most frightening event a person can experience in his or her lifetime. Despite the fact that many patients recover from their disease and go on to live healthy and normal lives, the big "C" word still feels like a death sentence to those who get the news.

There are standard tests and screenings that are currently used to detect cancer and make a diagnosis. Unfortunately, the nature of these tests often induces anxiety due to their invasiveness and the time it takes to analyze results. On the bright side, there is new and exciting research being done to develop tests that are less invasive and more accurate. They include liquid biopsies, breath, and saliva tests.

Detecting cancer early increases the chances of a successful outcome. That's why it's important for patients to be educated and recognize symptoms and signs that may suggest cancer at its earliest onset. And from there, to seek clarification through checkups to confirm or rule out cancer.

It's important to be your own best advocate. By becoming informed you can help yourself and your loved ones to seek help early. In this chapter, we provide an overview of standard and cutting edge diagnostic technologies, including preventive screenings that will one day become common place.

Medical Imaging Is Standard Practice

Medical imaging tests that use nuclear medicine are used to confirm or diagnose a condition. They allow your doctor to see what's going on inside of your body and help diagnose the cause of any issues. Examples of imaging tests are:

- X-rays
- Ultrasounds
- Mammography
- Computed tomography scan (CT)
- Magnetic resonance imaging (MRI)
- Nuclear scans

For example, virtual colonoscopy uses CT scans instead of a scope to detect abnormal growth both on the surface and below, within the intestines. The benefit of this is the avoidance of general anesthesia and accidental intestinal perforation. The downside is radiation exposure and the need for polyp removal, if present via colonoscopy.

Looking Inside the Body with a Video Camera

Endoscopy is a non-surgical medical procedure where a long, thin, flexible tube with a camera at the end is inserted into the body through an opening, such as your mouth or a small incision in the body, to observe an organ or tissue. It can be used to view the:

- Gastrointestinal tract (endoscopy, colonoscopy)
- Respiratory system (bronchoscopy)
- Heart and cardiovascular system (angiogram)
- Female reproductive system (laparoscopy)
- Urinary tract (cystoscopy)

It is often used to take a sample of a suspicious tissue so it can be analyzed for cancerous cells, this procedure is called a biopsy.

Look for innovative and non-invasive tests that may one day replace the need for frequent colonoscopies.

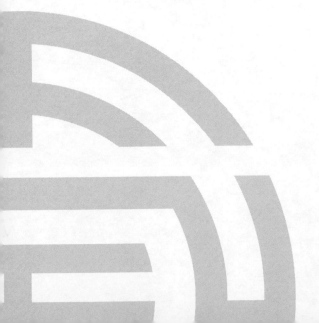

Cytology Tests Analyze Cells in Bodily Fluids

Cytology is a test where a sample of bodily fluids (blood, urine, plasma, etc.) is collected and viewed under a microscope. It looks for any abnormal shape or size in the cells examined that may indicate cancerous changes.

A normal cell should stay in the same area of its origin, but cancer cells travel or metastasize through blood and lymph vessels into a distant part of the body. For example, breast cells should only be found in the breasts, and not be found in the fluid of the lungs when it is collected for analysis. Often, when a cytology test is positive, a more invasive biopsy will follow.

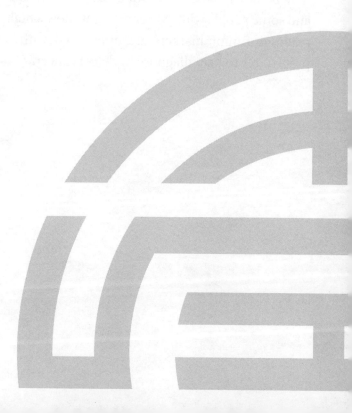

Tumor Markers Indicate Protein Levels Produced by Cancer

Tumor markers are proteins or other substances that are produced by cancer cells or normal cells in response to cancer or other non-cancerous conditions. Markers appear in blood, urine, or other body tissues. Some common examples are:

- CA-125 in ovarian cancer
- PSA (prostate-specific antigen) in prostate cancer
- CEA (carcino-embryonic antigen) in colon, gastrointestinal, breast, lung, and pancreatic cancer.

There are over 20 tumor markers.

An elevated tumor marker level can indicate cancer, but there may be other causes too. Not every cancer has a tumor marker and some people with cancer may not show a high tumor marker reading. Tumor markers are often used with other tests and procedures to help diagnose or detect cancer.

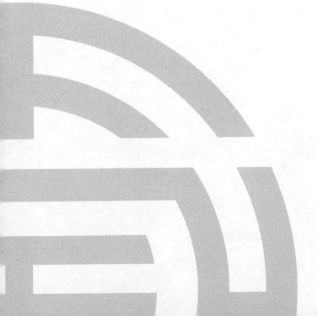

Circulating Tumor DNAs Is a Noninvasive and Complementary Diagnostic Test

Researchers from Johns Hopkins Kimmel Cancer Center have been exploring an approach sometimes referred to as liquid biopsies. Liquid biopsies could potentially complement or, in some cases, serve as an alternative to tissue biopsies. The approach relies on detecting bits of tumor material, known as circulating tumor DNAs (ctDNAs), that are found in blood or urine. The test is called CancerSeek and screens for eight cancer proteins at the same time, specifically:

- Ovary
- Liver
- Stomach
- Pancreas
- Esophagus
- Colorectal
- Lung
- Breast

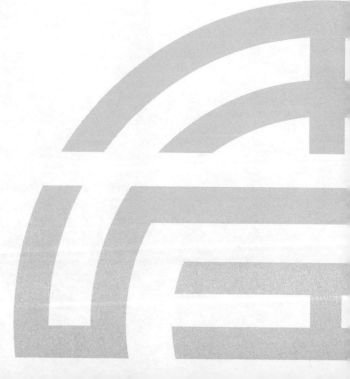

Liquid Biopsies for Early Detection of Certain Cancers

One potential application of ctDNA-based liquid biopsies is for detecting cancer in its early stages, when treatment may be most successful. In several studies liquid biopsy tests detected ctDNA in blood samples months before patients were diagnosed with cancer by traditional methods. The National Cancer Institute seems to agree stating, "there are liquid biopsy technologies that can noninvasively identify the presence of genetic material from cancer cells in the blood or molecular markers in urine or saliva that can identify precursor lesions or cancer at its earliest stages."

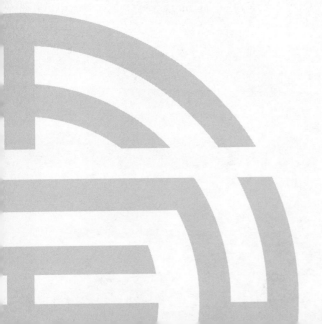

Monitoring Cancer Development During Treatment

Liquid biopsy tests have the added advantage of providing molecular information about cancer, which can change during and after treatment. For example, liquid biopsies could be used to monitor cancer development, track a patient's response to treatment, or as a "surveillance" method for people who have completed treatment but are at high risk of their disease returning.

Ask your doctor about liquid biopsy tests to monitor your progress during your cancer treatment period.

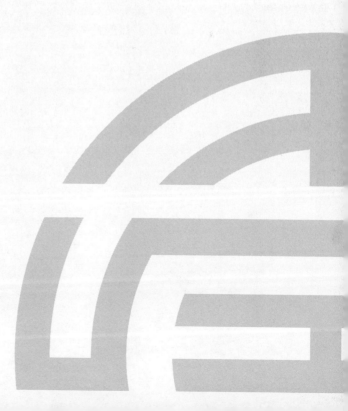

Taking Pieces of Suspicious Tissue via Biopsy

A biopsy involves surgically removing a small amount of tissue or a group of cells from a particular part of the body or organ. These cells are then analyzed for a diagnosis.

Biopsies, however, are not without risks. For example, the surgical site may bleed excessively or it can potentially spread cancer cells along the extraction route. Currently, less invasive ways to retrieve information from organs and tumors are being developed. For example, the liquid biopsy we mentioned earlier, or using a blood sample.

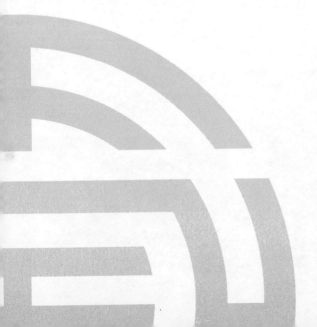

A Breath Test May Reveal Lung and Breast Cancers

Your breath can reveal many clues about your health, and not just what you had for dinner last night. The air that you breathe out contains many different chemicals called volatile organic compounds (VOCs). Studies have shown that exhaled breath from people with lung and breast cancers have a distinct odor signature of VOCs compared to the breath of people without such cancers.

In a breath test, you just breathe out and sensors in the equipment pick up your unique "breath signature." The VOCs in the breath sample are captured by the sensors and change colors when exposed to specific chemicals. The test could be as simple as a urine or saliva dipstick. Look out for its availability.

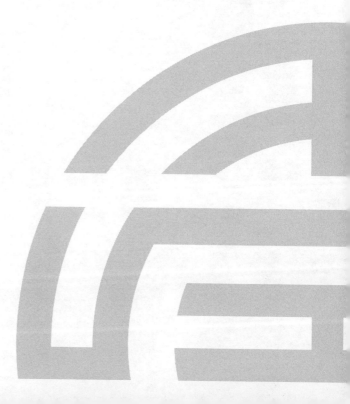

Saliva Tests May Shed Light on Early Stage Pancreatic Cancer

A simple swab of saliva may help diagnose early pancreatic cancer. Research presented at the American Society of Microbiology found people with pancreatic cancer have different types of bacteria in their saliva compared to those without. This is particularly good news since pancreatic cancer often goes undetected until it is at an advanced stage. Ask your doctor about its availability.

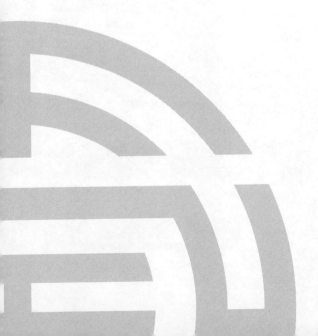

Stool DNA Tests May One Day Replace Colonoscopies

Wouldn't it be easier if a stool screening test for colorectal cancer could replace having to undergo a colonoscopy? Now, an easy-to-use stool test called Cologuard has been approved by the FDA to detect abnormal DNA changes and red blood cells.

Current screening guidelines do not eliminate the need for a traditional colonoscopy. However, experts agree that fecal DNA tests expand the testing options for colorectal cancer detection and may one day reduce the frequency of colonoscopies.

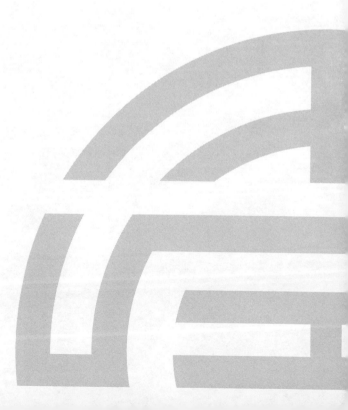

Cell-Free DNA Detects Cancer at Different Stages

Another new and noninvasive blood test called cell-free DNA (cfDNA) may someday detect numerous types of cancer at different stages with high precision. The test is not dependent on tumor cells or proteins produced by cancer cells, thus the name cell-free DNA. Instead, it looks at the gene activity of DNA to assess the development of cancer.

The ability of cfDNA evaluation to detect a wide range of cancer types at various stages suggests it could become a screening test for multiple cancers. Current research is focused on developing a generalized screening test, similar to a wellness exam, for the public.

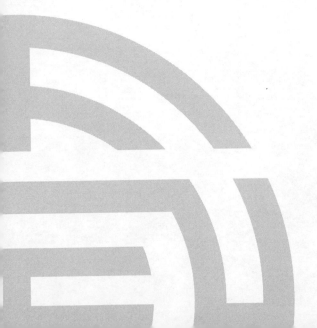

Genetic Test for Inherited Cancers

There are more than 1,000 genetic tests available for genetic disorders, such as cystic fibrosis, hemophilia, or Down syndrome. Predictive genetic tests are a type of test used to look for inherited gene mutations that might put a person at risk. It is an especially helpful tool for people with a family history of cancer. This is because they are often at a higher risk of developing cancer due to inherited mutations. For instance, if you have a family history of breast cancer, testing for BRCA mutations can identify if you are predisposed to developing breast and ovarian cancer. Less than 15% of all cancer is due to inherited genetics though, so there's no need to panic.

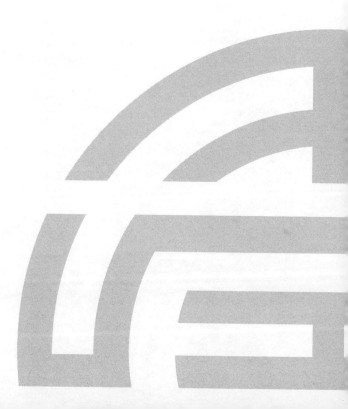

Do Not Ignore Chronic, Persistent Cough

Acute cough or blood-tinged saliva usually is due to simple infections like bronchitis or sinusitis. However, anyone with a nagging cough that lasts more than a month and gets worse should see a doctor. This is especially true if there is blood in the mucus, chest pain that's worse when coughing, and shortness of breath. Your doctor may order an X-ray or CT scan to rule out pneumonia or, in a worst case scenario, cancer of the lung, head, and neck.

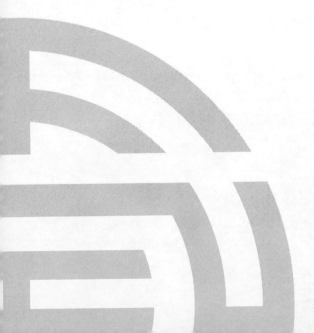

Be on the Lookout for Unexpected Weight Loss

Sudden weight loss that is unexpected and unexplained can happen due to many diseases. However, sudden, unexplained weight loss of 10 pounds or more may be the first sign of cancer.

Cancer cells, not unlike those in an adolescent teenager's body, grow rapidly. These cells require massive amounts of energy and often divert nutrients away from healthy cells, therefore causing sudden weight loss. Go see a doctor if you or someone you know experiences such symptoms.

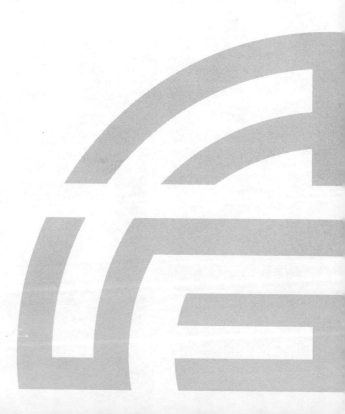

Take Unexplained Loss of Appetite Seriously

Hunger is normal in healthy individuals. As one ages, his or her body releases less and less gastric juices, which can affect one's appetite. That's why the elderly tend to have smaller appetites compared to when they were young. Certain medications can interfere with one's appetite too.

However, if your appetite suddenly drops without warning, especially with accompanying weight loss, it is a reason for concern. This may be a warning sign of stomach, pancreatic, colon, or ovarian cancer. These cancers put pressure on the digestive organs and make you feel too full to eat. A study actually showed that cancer produces a substance called MIC-1 that promotes weight loss by suppressing appetite. When you find difficulty eating even your favorite foods, be sure to have a health checkup.

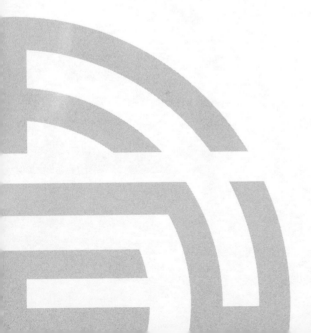

Look Ma, I'm Bleeding

It's never a good sign if you start bleeding for no reason.

If blood is coughed or vomited up it may indicate lung, esophageal, stomach, or oral cancers. Blood in the stool may be due to hemorrhoids or colorectal cancer, although it is usually detected via a stool test since stool blood is normally not visible to the naked eye. Blood in urine may indicate bladder cancer or prostate cancer in men.

Vaginal bleeding between menses may indicate polyps, fibroid, cysts, and cancer of the uterus, ovary, and cervix. Do not ignore your regular Pap smear which detects cervical cancer.

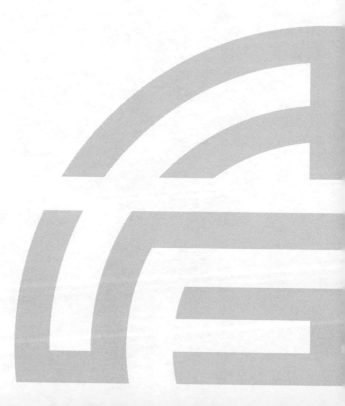

Sudden Changes in Bowel Habit
Is a Cause for Alarm

If you haven't changed your diet but your bowel habits change, sit up and pay attention. When your normally log-like stool become pencil-thin, this may be due to a lesion partially obstructing the rectal passageway. Occasionally, colon cancer can cause continuous diarrhea and at other times unusual constipation. Some people may feel as if they need to have a bowel movement and are not relieved of the feeling even after they have had it. A significant change in bowel habits that cannot be easily explained by dietary changes needs to be evaluated. If any of these abnormal bowel complaints last more than a week, be sure to see your doctor.

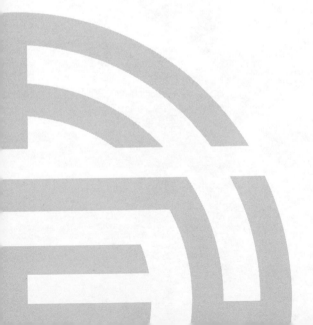

Urinary Changes May Signal More Serious Problems

If your urinating habits suddenly change for no reason, you should pay attention. Particularly, if you are frequently urinating, have small and slow volume and flow, or if there's blood in your urine you should see a doctor immediately. Chances are you are suffering from a urinary tract or bladder infection. If the changes are accompanied by lower back pain, the affliction may be in the kidneys.

Most men will suffer from harmless prostate enlargement as they age and will often have these urinary symptoms. However, these symptoms can also signal prostate cancer. A prostate MRI may be ordered and, if the results necessitate, biopsies performed.

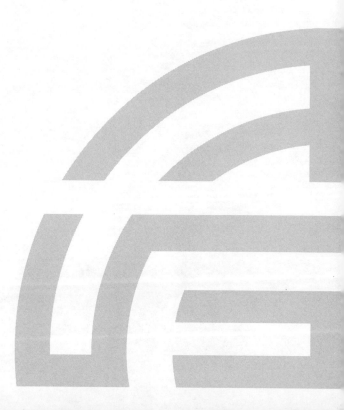

Are You Anemic for No Reason?

Anemia is a condition where a person has a lower than normal red blood cell count. There are many types of anemia, but blood loss almost always causes iron deficiency anemia. Unless there is an obvious source of ongoing blood loss, this anemia needs to be investigated.

Many cancers can cause anemia, but colorectal cancers most commonly cause iron deficiency anemia. Your doctor may order a colonoscopy, endoscopy, and CT scans of your upper and lower intestinal tracts.

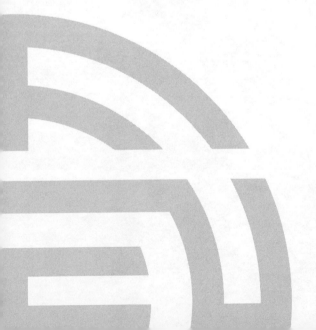

Do Not Ignore Persistent Pain

Pain that doesn't go away requires immediate medical attention. Naturally, there are many causes of pain that aren't cancer, ranging from injuries and infections, to ulcers and obstructions. However, cancer can cause pain, and in some cancers such as bone and testicular pain comes at the start of the condition. Pain can appear in different places and different ways. For instance, as tumors grow they can push into other organs or areas in the body, displacing an organ or compressing a nerve as they metastasize. This can lead to headaches, chest, abdominal, back, and bone pain.

Other examples are:

- Back pain which could be coming from a tumor that has metastasized from colon, prostate, ovarian, liver, or rectal cancer.
- Chest pain that radiates into the shoulder or arm can be a sign of a lung tumor, breast cancer, or lymphoma.
- Pain and distention in the pelvic region could be a sign of ovarian cancer.
- Headaches and sudden vision or hearing loss can be due to a brain tumor.

Night Sweats May Mean More Than Midlife Change

Sweating is your body's natural way of regulating temperature. Excessive sweating at night can be caused by hormonal changes in both men and women during midlife menopausal or andropausal changes. Additionally, certain medications such as prednisone and psychotropic drugs can induce night sweats.

However, when night sweats are accompanied by other symptoms such as fever, nose bleeds, or unexpected weight loss it can be an early sign of certain cancers. Talk to your doctor about your night sweats if other symptoms are present.

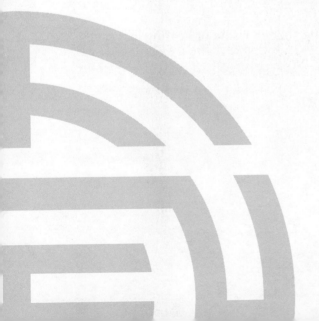

Lumps in the Body Are Not Just Fat

There are all kinds of lumps one encounters in life, but it's the lumps you find in your body that you need to worry about. While many lumps are benign, fibrous ones or fluid-filled lumps like cysts should be kept an eye on. If lumps appear in breasts, testicles, or lymph node areas such as the armpits, groin, and neck you need to get them examined by your doctor.

Usually, lymph nodes swollen due to infection will shrink within a month, but if it remains it is a good reason to get it checked out. After imaging tests, if the lumps appear suspicious a biopsy will follow to rule out cancer. Remember, early detection means a better outcome, if it is in fact cancer.

Track Skin Changes with Regular Photographs

As you get older your skin seems to grow more protuberances, like that of an ancient rock. Yes, it's true, and you're not alone. Aging skin, longer sun exposure, and declining immunity all cause skin cell changes that can lead to skin cancer.

Be observant about obvious changes in a wart or mole. Multi-colored moles that have irregular edges, bleed, enlarge or darken in color may be cancerous. Sores that don't heal could be a warning. People's memories are generally not reliable, therefore it's wise to track changes in your skin growth by taking pictures regularly.

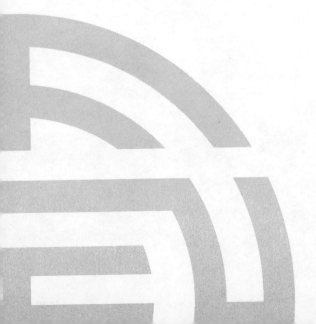

Do You Have Chronic Indigestion or Difficulty Swallowing?

A vast number of people suffer from chronic heartburn without it leading to serious problems. However, chronic, untreated gastro-esophageal reflux disorder (GERD) may lead to Barrett esophagus, which in turn can lead to esophageal cancer. Sometimes the symptoms can include difficulty swallowing, coughing, or hoarseness. Regular endoscopic exams can monitor the progression of your GERD and, if necessary, a biopsy can be done to rule out suspicious lesions.

Naturally, prevention is achievable by avoiding certain foods, such as:

- Red meat
- Acidic foods
- Spicy foods
- Deep fried foods
- Rich foods
- Alcohol
- Coffee

One can also heal the gut lining with herbs and supplements.

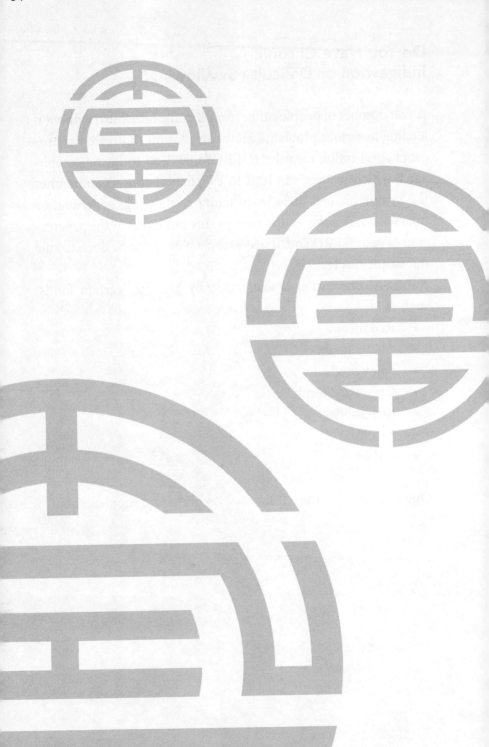

Chapter 4:
Integrative Cancer Care
with Chinese Medicine

Imagine a world in which medicine was oriented toward healing rather than disease, where doctors believed in the natural healing capacity of human beings and emphasized prevention above treatment. In such a world, doctors and patients would be partners working toward the same ends.

—Andrew Weil

People throughout the world use a variety of strategies to cope with the physical, emotional, and spiritual impact of cancer. One strategy that has emerged in recent years is integrative oncology. It is a scientific discipline that focuses on combining conventional and complementary cancer treatments to address the diverse needs of cancer patients and their families. Many complementary therapies originated outside of North America thousands of years ago and are still practiced often in their countries of origin. Examples include acupuncture, yoga, and herbal medicine. In China, the use of Traditional Chinese Medicine (TCM) herbal therapies for cancer patients exceeds 80%.

The history of Chinese medicine and its approach to cancer dates back more than 3,000 years. It is mentioned in the Yellow Emperor's Classic of Medicine, one of the most esteemed and earliest written medical books in China, and possibly in the world. As early as the 11th century BC, descriptions of tumors were inscribed on animal bones and bamboo tablets. Some physicians specialized in wai ke, or external medicine, and took care of these lesions. Lesions were referred to as liu, meaning tumor, and derived from a word meaning accumulation and stagnation. Around the 2nd century BC, tumors became known as hard lumps or ulcerated lesions. Both benign and malignant tumors were further differentiated as ulcers, abscesses, carbuncles, or hard lumps. Since the 12th century AD, the term ai was used exclusively to describe cancer.

Chinese medicine's approach to disease differs from Western medicines. In Chinese medicine, disease is thought of as an imbalance of the whole person. It takes into account changing environmental and emotional factors which may affect the manifestation and progression of the disease. The goal of Chinese medicine is to restore balance to the body. This is done using:

- Acupuncture
- Bodywork
- Herbal and nutritional therapies
- Qigong
- Meditation

The treatment works to rid infection, nourish life force (qi) and blood, eliminate toxins from the body, increase circulation, and restore the balance of yin and yang in the body and organ systems. In the case of cancer, Chinese medicine seeks to strengthen patient's resistance to disease while eliminating toxins from the body. This approach is called fu zheng qu xie, or simply Fu Zheng therapy.

Chinese medicine's reputation as a complementary treatment has grown in the United States over the last 20 years. Since 2006, the Office of Cancer Complementary and Alternative Medicine

(OCCAM) has hosted regular international conferences with cancer researchers and oncologists from the United States, Canada, China, South Korea, Australia, Taiwan, Singapore, and Hong Kong. These conferences promote collaboration between the National Cancer Institute (NCI) and various institutes in China. They also have enhanced the dialogue and understanding between Chinese and Western medical systems on cancer prevention, treatment, and symptom management.

These joint efforts have allowed scientists and clinicians from both countries to research the ingredients in Chinese herbal medicine. This allows them to look for potential anti-cancer applications either alone or in combination with Western medicine. The anti-cancer mechanisms and actions of certain herbal medicines have been eliminated through such collaborative settings. There have been a tremendous amount of studies on Chinese medicine and cancer. A search of PubMed, NIH's archive of published studies, yielded more than 20,000 publications on Chinese medicine and cancer since 1990.

Patients with cancer often use methods such as acupuncture, meditation, herbs, and dietary supplements in addition to their conventional cancer treatment. In 2003, the establishment of the Society of Integrative Oncology (SIO) helped further legitimize the term "integrative oncology." The definition of integrative oncology states:

Integrative oncology is a patient-centered, evidence-informed field to cancer care that utilizes mind-body therapies, natural products, and lifestyle modifications from different traditions alongside conventional cancer treatments. Integrative oncology aims to optimize health, quality of life, and clinical outcomes across the cancer care continuum and to empower people to prevent cancer and become active participants in their care before, during and beyond cancer treatment.

In the US, major cancer centers had already taken the lead in integrating Chinese and Western medicine for cancer care. For example, the Memorial Sloan Kettering Cancer Center in New York City established its Integrative Medicine Service as early as 1999. Soon after, MD Anderson Cancer Center in Houston and the Dana-Farber Cancer Center in Boston formed dedicated programs focused on integrating complementary therapies into cancer care. Over the past decade, the presence of integrative medicine at US National Cancer Institute centers has increased greatly, with the majority of centers now offering some form of integrative treatment.

In the following pages of this chapter we will introduce various modalities of Chinese medicine. As well as showing why, based on strong scientific evidence, they should be an essential part of your integrative cancer treatment program.

Acupuncture May Be the Only Successful Therapy for Certain Symptoms

The acceptance of acupuncture as a viable treatment for cancer symptoms has risen. Consequently, this gives recognition that it may be the only successful therapy in many circumstances. For instance, a patient with pruritus, or intense itching, enjoyed relief for their last days of life following acupuncture. Other cases of acupuncture helping include a patient with terminal esophageal cancer enjoying a full night's sleep, patients with post-chemo neuralgia having less pain and requiring fewer medications, and post stomach surgery patients finding relief from nausea and vomiting when antiemetic drugs had no effect.

According to Peter A.S. Johnstone, MD of Moffitt Cancer Center, a leading NCI-designated cancer center in Florida, "There seems no doubt that acupuncture should no longer be considered a 'complementary' therapy in the milieu of cancer symptom management; our task now is to fashion mechanisms for our patients to avail themselves of the opportunity. In the past 10 years acupuncture has, rightly, become included in major journals, tumor board discussions, and medical staff privileges. The near future promises more success."

Ask your doctor or a trusted friend for a referral to a licensed acupuncturist and Chinese medicine practitioner, or see the Resources section for professional referrals.

Most Patients in China Use Chinese Medicine for Cancer Therapy

It may sound obvious, but the use of Traditional Chinese medicine by cancer patients in China is exceptionally high. According to a study published in Evidence-Based Complementary and Alternative Medicine, 83% of patients used Chinese medicine at the same time as their modern cancer treatments. Chinese herbal medicine and nutrition were the most used, followed by qi gong, tai chi, and acupuncture. 63% of patients notified their oncologist about their Chinese medicine use, and physicians were generally supportive. The most common reason for use was to improve immune function and quality of life. Chinese herbal medicine was often used with the goal of enhancing cancer treatment, a use that over half of oncologists agreed with.

The good news is that you don't have to travel all the way to China to receive the same integrative approach to cancer care. There are licensed practitioners of acupuncture and Chinese medicine in the US who have been trained in integrative oncology. They offer high quality and effective protocols to increase quality of life, reduce side effects of cancer treatments, and, in some cases, prolong survival time.

Acupressure Relieves Nausea and Vomiting

The use of acupressure is based on acupuncture meridian theory. The theory is that when an acupoint is stimulated along certain meridians it activates the body's innate self-healing and relief response. Meridians are energy pathways that transport qi throughout the body. A review of 23 studies published in the Journal of Pain and Symptom Management found that a daily nine-minute acupressure treatment given prior to chemotherapy decreased nausea and vomiting. The treatment began on the first day of chemotherapy and continued for 21 days, and the benefits were seen between days 2 to 11.

To get a similar effect yourself, simply apply steady pressure with your thumb on the acupoint P6 (or neiguan, as it's known in Chinese) located about 2 inches above the crease of the wrist on either arm. You will find it in-between two tendons that become pronounced when making a fist.

Alternatively, there are devices on the market with trade names like Sea Band and Motion Sickness Relief Band that are similarly effective.

What You Eat Matters When it Comes to Cancer

Many studies have identified the anti-cancer properties of certain foods. For example, an Asian style, plant based diet has been shown to vastly lower one's lifetime cancer risk.

Other studies have discovered foods that either directly lead to cancer or contribute to increased cancer risks. Western style diets heavy in red meat, sugar, saturated fats, and smoked or barbecued meat lead to more cancer incidence, especially that of colorectal cancers.

More often than not, chemotherapy causes intense gastric distress that leads to nausea, vomiting, low appetite, and stomach pain. The result is that most cancer patients lose weight, strength, and energy during their treatment. This can sometimes end their treatments prematurely. Neither outcome is desirable.

This can be avoided though. During our 30-plus years working with oncologists, we have found that eating more high quality protein and good fats during cancer treatments can prevent weight loss. This diet also helped maintain healthy red blood cell and platelet levels. However, after cancer treatment is over, we advocate a predominantly plant-based diet to reduce recurrence. This is also a great idea for those who are interested in cancer prevention, in general. We also counsel our patients on tailoring their diet according to their Elemental Body Type. See Chapter 5 for more advice on diet and nutrition.

Acupuncture Proven Safe and Effective

Acupuncture is a common and effective treatment for a number of cancer symptoms, including chemotherapy-induced nausea and vomiting. In the integrative oncology setting, acupuncture and Traditional Chinese Medicine have become more recognized. Many oncology clinics, academic health centers, and comprehensive cancer centers recommend and administer acupuncture treatment. The most recent research demonstrates that acupuncture is safe, tolerable, and effective for a range of side effects resulting from conventional cancer treatments.

Ask your doctor or a trusted friend for a referral to a licensed acupuncturist and Chinese medicine practitioner, or see the Resources section for professional referrals.

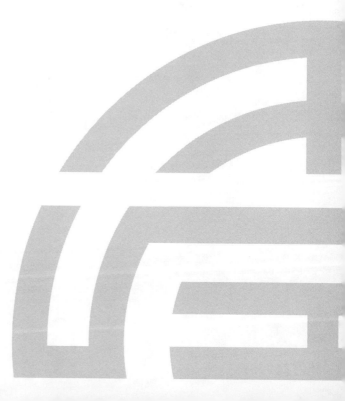

A Majority of People Around the World Use Complementary Medicine

The integration of conventional and traditional medicine is increasing in prevalence around the world. A review of studies performed in Europe, North America, Australia, and New Zealand found that the use of complementary medicines has been increasing, with almost half of cancer patients reporting use in the present-day. This prevalence is likely to be much higher in other parts of the world. For instance, an estimated 71% of the population of Chile and 65% of the population in rural India use traditional medicine to help meet their primary health care needs.

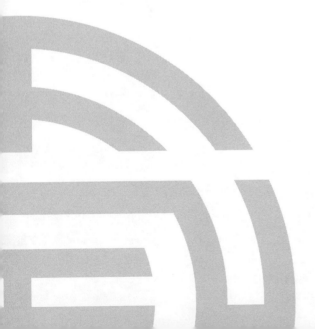

Chinese Herbal Therapy Improved Survival for Advanced Colorectal Cancer

Researchers were curious whether the use of Chinese herbal therapy made any difference in the survival rate for advanced cancer. These researchers conducted a study of patients in China who had undergone surgery for stage II and III colorectal cancer and received comprehensive conventional treatments. Follow-up visits were conducted over five years, comparing patients who used Chinese herbal therapy for more than one year versus those who used little or none. The conclusion by the researchers was that, "longer duration of Chinese herbal use is associated with improved survival outcomes in stage II and III colorectal cancer patients."

The best results from Chinese herbal therapy are achieved by consulting doctors of Chinese medicine who are well versed in herb-drug interaction and can individualize an herbal formula or protocol specific to each patient's needs. Always inform your doctor before beginning any new health and fitness regimen.

Acupuncture Relieves Cancer Pain and Chemo-Induced Neuropathy

Cancer-related pain is one of the most common but difficult symptoms to manage. It is reported that more than 50% of patients with cancer experience pain. Cancer pain frequently occurs at different stages of the cancer journey:

- 25% in newly diagnosed patients.
- 33% in patients receiving anti-cancer treatment.
- Up to 75% in later stage cancers.

In a trial, patients with chronic neuropathic pain following cancer therapy were treated with auricular acupuncture, a treatment using acupoints exclusively in the ear. The results showed that the acupuncture group experienced a 36% reduction in pain intensity, whereas those without had a 2% reduction. A study on patients with peripheral neuropathy showed that 83% of those treated with acupuncture had improved nerve conduction. Whereas those without acupuncture only had a 20% reduction. A recent study of multiple myeloma patients with moderate to severe chemo-induced neuropathy had significantly reduced pain and improved function following 10 weeks of acupuncture treatment.

When receiving acupuncture treatments for neuropathy, be sure to ask your licensed acupuncturist to add electrostimulation (a mild electrical current) for enhanced symptom relief.

Leading US Cancer Centers Increasingly Offer Integrative Medicine Content and Services

Cancer centers have increased their integrative medicine therapies in response to their patients' unmet needs. Researchers conducted a review of 45 NCI-designated cancer center websites and found that between 2009 and 2016 there was a significant increase in the number of websites mentioning acupuncture, dance therapy, healing touch, hypnosis, massage, meditation, qi gong, and yoga. In fact, the most common integrative therapies mentioned on the websites were exercise, acupuncture, and meditation. These were followed by yoga, massage, and music therapy. The majority of the websites also provided information on nutrition, dietary supplements, and herbal therapy. The most common therapies offered were:

- Acupuncture/massage
- Meditation/yoga
- Nutrition consultation
- Dietary supplements consultation
- Herb consultation

Sometimes family members and friends have to advocate for a patient by asking for integrative medical services onsite, or if not available referrals to qualified professionals.

Chinese Herbal Relief for Joint Pain from Aromatase Inhibitor Drugs

Patients with estrogen-receptor positive (ER+) breast cancer take estrogen-blocking drugs like Tamoxifen and other aromatase inhibitor (AI) drugs to suppress and block estrogen that is triggering cancer cell proliferation. The most common side effects of these drugs, besides other menopausal symptoms, is muscle and joint pain. At the moment, there is no suitable treatment in conventional medicine for some patients with this debilitating condition. This is because long term use of non-steroidal anti-inflammatory drugs (NSAIDs) or opioids come with unacceptable side effects. As a result, up to 20% of patients stop their AI treatments due to decreased quality of life.

There is now effective relief for AI-induced pain. A Chinese herbal formula is being used in the Beijing Cancer Hospital for breast cancer patients suffering from muscle and joint pain due to aromatase inhibitor drugs. Its efficacy has been confirmed in a study published in the journal Breast. The study involved the Chinese herbal formula code named YSJG. YSJG contains rehmannia, cuscuta, cypress, ligustici, corydalis, trachelospermum, and other herbs. Patients treated with YSJG granules showed significant pain reduction after 12 and 24 weeks. Improvements in physical, social/family, emotional, and functional well-being were seen as well. Moreover, YSJG granules did not increase serum estradiol levels. This is desirable since the goal of treatment is to suppress and block estrogen because a majority of breast cancer cases in North America are due to excess estrogen in the body.

The results of this study demonstrate that YSJG granules are effective, safe, and well-tolerated in managing AI-induced muscle and joint pain.

Inquire with doctors of Chinese medicine who are familiar with and are able to replicate the formula used in this study. See the Resources section for professional referrals as well as sources for the YSJG formula.

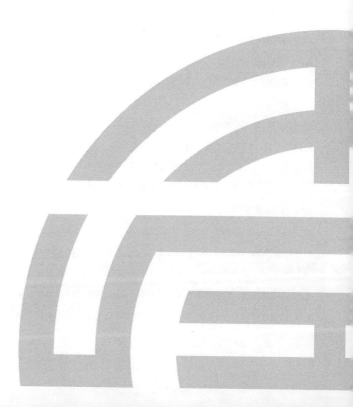

Qi Gong Positively Impacts Well-Being for Cancer Patients

Major cancer centers in the US are increasingly offering qi gong. It is a mind-body practice, which originated from China, and has been found to improve well-being in cancer patients. Qi gong helps:

- Mood
- Fatigue
- Pain
- Inflammation
- Cognitive function
- Immune function
- High blood pressure
- Diabetes
- Insomnia

A number of studies have shown that regular qi gong practice has the potential to improve cancer-related quality of life, and is directly linked to cancer prevention and survival.

A study published in the Annals of Oncology showed that practicing qi gong along with usual care improved the quality of life (QOL) of cancer patients. The finding was discovered at a 10-week follow-up. Participants who completed the qi gong practice total QOL scores were significantly improved compared to the usual care control group. Another significant finding from this study was the positive effects of qi gong on inflammation, which was evidenced by the drop in the inflammation marker C-Reactive Protein (CRP). The result was significantly less cancer-related fatigue and better total mood status. Specifically, the qi gong group had reduced tension, anxiety and depression, and increased vigor. Finally, no adverse effects of qi gong were reported by the cancer patients in this trial.

The Tao of Wellness collaborates with the Cancer Support Community in offering free qi gong classes for cancer patients and caretakers weekly at Saint John's Hospital in Santa Monica, California. There are qi gong classes offered in community centers throughout the US.

See Chapter 6 and Resources for more on qi gong.

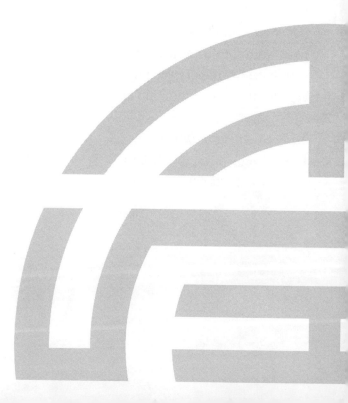

Tai Chi Enhances Immune Function, Balance, and Lowers Risks of Falls

To the Western world, familiar images of China include the Great Wall, the Forbidden City, and people in the parks moving gracefully, practicing tai chi. Tai chi and similar practices have existed in China for nearly five thousand years, and are part of the healing tradition of Chinese medicine. Health benefits of tai chi include enhanced immune function, better mood and blood pressure, and reduced pain and stiffness. It also improves proprioception—awareness of the position and movement of the body, which results in better balance and lowers the risk of falls.

Recent studies have indicated that tai chi enhances the immune system and relieves pain, anxiety, and stress in both cancer patients and survivors. According to Lorenzo Cohen, Ph.D. of MD Anderson Cancer Center, "In terms of the evidence that's out there and the scientific literature, practices such as Tai chi have been found to help improve patients' quality of life...can also have an impact on physiological functioning, improving aspects of immune function and decreasing stress hormones."

You can attend tai chi classes offered in community centers and fitness clubs throughout the US, as well as in some select yoga and martial arts studios.

Massage Improves Mood and Energy, Lowers Nausea and Pain

Massage is a beneficial complementary therapy for cancer patients. Most patients have reported that it reduced their anxiety and depression, lowered nausea and pain, and relieved them of the fatigue and stress associated with cancer and anti-cancer treatments like chemotherapy and radiation.

A review of trials involving massage for cancer patients has confirmed many of its benefits. The review found that massage provided cancer patients with reduced anxiety and depression, lowered nausea and pain, and it relieved them of fatigue. Massage also significantly reduced stress hormone, as measured by blood cortisol levels. A large study of 1,300 subjects concluded that, "Benefits of massage lasted longer in the patients who had the longer sessions compared with shorter, 20-minute sessions."

Massage and bodywork services can be found in the offices of integrative healthcare providers. These include acupuncturists, chiropractors, physical therapists, and sports medicine specialists, as well as stand-alone massage businesses. All massage therapists must be licensed by the city they practice in. Clinical and massage businesses' quality of service differ depending on whether the massage is "medical" or "feel-good," respectively. Clinical massage may also be covered by your health insurance. Check with your provider.

Aromatherapy/Essential Oil Benefits Sleep, Mood, and Well-Being

Essential oils have been around since the beginning of time. Throughout history, essential oils have been used to relieve symptoms, recover from illness, and help people sleep better, as well as feel more calm and alert. Essential oils are natural aromatic oils that contain terpenoids. Terpenoids are the volatile organic compounds that give each plant a distinct fragrance and flavor. They are found in various parts of plants, particularly the flowers, and have amazing medicinal properties.

Research on the use of aromatherapy/essential oils for cancer patients suggests a short-term benefit to reduce anxiety and depression, improve sleep, and increase overall wellbeing. This effect has been suggested to last up to 2 weeks and may be used safely by cancer patients. There is a considerable amount of published research on the anti-inflammatory, anti-oxidant, and anti-microbial activities of essential oils. Several preclinical trials are underway to explore the apoptosis inducing and anti-cancer effects of a number of essential oils.

You may add a few drops of essential oils to a diffuser so that its aromatic compounds are inhaled through the air. You can also apply it to your skin. If essential oils are applied directly to your skin, then they may need to be applied along with a carrier oil, such as olive oil or coconut oil. Try applying essential oils of lavender to soothe your anxiety and calm stress, peppermint to enhance mental alertness and boost energy, chamomile to help ensure a good night's sleep, or ginger to reduce nausea and vomiting.

Meditation Slows Cellular Aging and Reduces Symptoms

One of the major causes of cancer is aging. As cellular functions decline, more errors and less repairs occur as cells divide, this leads to mutations that can multiply into a tumor. One of the measurements for cellular aging is telomeres, the protein caps at the end of your chromosomes that determine how quickly a cell ages. A study published in the journal Cancer showed that telomeres stayed the same length in cancer survivors who meditated or took part in support groups over a three-month period. In comparison, the telomeres of cancer survivors who didn't participate in these groups shortened during the three-month study.

Research over the last 20 years has also found meditation to be helpful in relieving symptoms and improving the quality of life for people with cancer. Meditation was found to:
- Elevate mood
- Improve memory and focus
- Decrease depression and anxiety
- Reduce nausea
- Boost immune function

Best of all, it has no side effects whatsoever.

Refer to Chapter 6 for a simple, guided meditation for stress release and other meditation practices.

Fasting Reduces Insulin Resistance and Improves Response to Chemotherapy

The practice of fasting for health or spiritual purposes dates back to the beginning of human civilization. Chinese medicine has long advocated supervised fasting for restoring balance, and promoting health and longevity. The health benefits of fasting are now being validated with studies showing that it may help with cancer treatment. There is growing evidence that suggests that fasting helps fight cancer by lowering insulin resistance and levels of inflammation, as well as helping make cancer cells more responsive to chemotherapy while protecting other cells.

Fasting is defined as consumption of less than 200 calories each day, although abundant fluids are encouraged to prevent dehydration. It also induces autophagy, the breaking down of cells (i.e. cancer cells) for parts to be reused later. This process plays an important role in prevention and treatment of cancer.

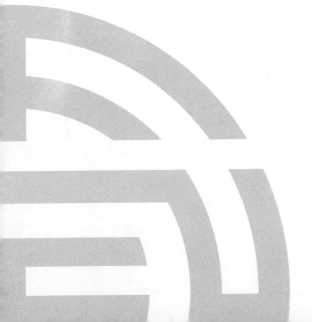

A review of 22 studies of fasting's effect on cancer showed substantially suppressed tumor progression, improved survival, and decreased chemotherapy side effects such as reduced bone marrow suppression. When fasting was paired with chemotherapy, the anti-tumor effects of chemotherapy drugs increased. The study outcomes suggested that fasting for 48 to 72 hours prior to chemotherapy was crucial for achieving the positive effects of fasting therapy. Although weight loss occurred during fasting, once normal food intake was reintroduced most participants weight returned to normal.

If you are interested in incorporating fasting into your anti-cancer program be sure to work with your integrative healthcare provider in order to coordinate close supervision.

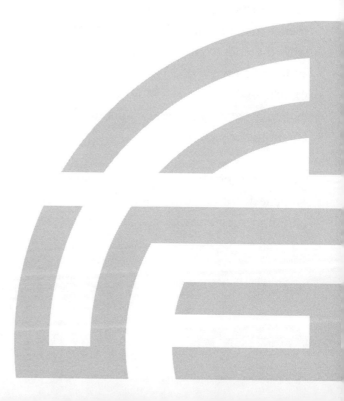

Antioxidants May Improve Tumor Response in Cancer Therapy

Many oncologists advise patients not to take vitamin supplements during their cancer therapy. This is due to fears that the use of vitamins like glutathione, vitamin C, and selenium may protect cancer cells from the destructive effects of chemotherapy. These vitamins exert antioxidant actions, and many oncologists fear they may counter oxidative stress and the damage to cancer cells that chemotherapy promotes. As it turns out, some of the risk may be more theory than fact.

A systematic review of studies from 1966 to 2007 found no evidence that antioxidant supplements interfered with chemotherapy. Additionally, some studies showed using antioxidants such as glutathione, vitamin C, and selenium may improve tumor response to treatment and survival rates. These supplements may also help protect normal cells without interfering with the effectiveness of cancer therapy antioxidants. Another systematic review of 33 studies found evidence that using antioxidants with chemotherapy resulted in less toxicity, while also assisting patients to better tolerate the side effects from their chemotherapy treatments.

Before starting any dietary supplement regimens, we advise that you check with a knowledgeable integrative healthcare provider and inform your oncologist about what you are taking.

Yoga Modulates Stress-Immune Response in Cancer Patients

Many cancer patients have found yoga to be helpful in promoting flexibility, muscle strength, and calmness. It has been practiced in China and India, where yoga originated, for thousands of years. In modern times, studies have shown that regularly practicing yoga resulted in a reduction in stress hormones, increased relaxation, and improved nervous system function. The stress reducing effect of yoga is particularly important in cancer patients who have a constant worry due to their disease.

Numerous studies of yoga have shown reductions in cortisol, inflammatory cytokines, and improved natural killer cell (NK) production. The reduction in cortisol (stress hormone) means reduced fatigue, improved sleep, and improvement in immune response. Yoga is known to modulate psycho-neuro-endocrine, which is the interaction between the mind, nervous system, and hormonal system. It also helps the psycho-neuro-immune axis, or interaction between the mind, nervous system, and immune function. In other words, regularly practicing yoga restores balance to all of the systems in the body that are critical to fighting cancer.

You can find yoga classes in community recreation centers, fitness clubs, and yoga studios. You can also take classes online and streamed via the internet. Be sure to check with your healthcare provider before beginning any new health and fitness regimen.

Integrating Acupuncture into Palliative Cancer Care

Oncology acupuncture is a new specialty. It has become a promising field of research due to more and more cancer patients seeking non-pharmacological alternatives for symptom management. While different reasons have been suggested to explain its efficacy, its role has become that of alleviating the side effects induced by chemotherapy or radiation treatment.

In a paper published in the Journal of Traditional and Complementary Medicine, the authors reviewed hundreds of studies on acupuncture for cancer symptom relief. They found that acupuncture was effective in relieving:

- Hot flashes
- Xerostomia (mouth ulcers) induced by radiation treatments
- Nausea and vomiting from chemotherapy
- Cancer pain
- Fatigue
- Insomnia

Seek out licensed acupuncturists who have graduated from an accredited university and who have undertaken additional training in oncology acupuncture. You should avoid health professionals who do "dry needling," or completed a mere weekend course in acupuncture. Your health and wellbeing deserves highly experienced and effective practitioners.

Chapter 5: What You Eat — Diet, Nutrition, and Supplements

Let food be thy medicine and medicine be thy food.

—Hippocrates

What you eat matters, especially during cancer treatments. This chapter will cover what to eat to help prevent cancer recurring or ever occurring at all. We will also address the unique dietary needs of cancer patients going through treatment and how to manage the side effects that often come with it.

Epigenetics has given us a new understanding of diet and nutrition. Epigenetics focuses on studying how genes get turned on or off with nutrients. In other words, how does what you're eating affect your cells. The study examines nutrients that can stop potential tumor cells, help tumor suppressor genes, and mob up free radicals.

Research on the body's microorganisms and their role in immunity has revealed important bacteria living in the intestines. These good bacteria need the right fermented foods in order to keep gut immunity running at 100%.

The relationship between diet and cancer is supported when you look at the variation of cancer around the world. For instance, one study showed that Asians that move to the West raise their cancer risk ten to twenty five times. This is in part due to the major shift that happens to their diet. In this chapter, we will show you why diet is fundamental to slow aging and prevent cancer.

Many recent studies have confirmed the wisdom shared by Hippocrates, Chinese physicians, and other medical traditions throughout the ages: "Food is the best medicine, and the best medicine is food." It's no surprise that what you eat is linked to your risk of getting cancer. That said, there is no ultimate anti-cancer diet that will work for everyone. No two people are the same, and everyone has their varying needs. Nevertheless, a plant-based diet is still considered to be the gold standard to prevent cancer. The most important principle of Chinese medicine is that the most effective healing method is a personalized one. This means taking into account each person's constitution, gender, age, illness, psycho-spiritual, geographic, and seasonal needs. This principle is expressed through every treatment modality in Chinese medicine.

This chapter looks at how to find out your specific needs and what foods will meet those needs. By accomplishing specific health criteria, you decrease your chance of developing cancer. In the coming pages, we will tell you about foods with anti-cancer properties and nutritional supplements that work to prevent cancer. Finally, we share with you our Tao of Wellness Cancer Nutrition Program. We have provided this to thousands of patients over the last 30 years, it integrates the wisdom of Chinese medicine and the science of Western nutrition to support patients before, during, and beyond cancer treatments.

Eat for Your Element—Personalizing Your Diet

Chinese medicine recognizes the unique differences in all people. It categorizes these differences into five main personality and body types called the Five Elements–Wood, Fire, Earth, Metal, and Water. Each person has a core Element and reflects the character strengths and health vulnerabilities of it. That is why it's beneficial to eat according to one's element.

You can discover your Five Element personality and constitution by taking a short online quiz at infinichi.com, or refer to Chapter 7.

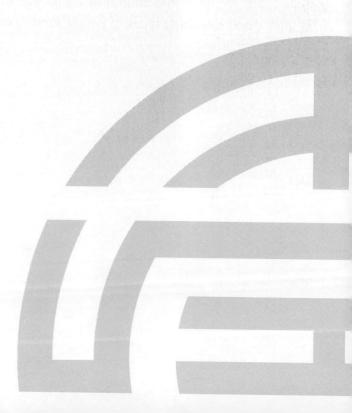

Wood Element Diet and Nutrition

Of all the elemental types, a Wood person is the most vulnerable to toxins. It is in one's best interest to severely limit or completely eliminate alcohol, cigarettes, recreational drugs, most pain relievers, and caffeine. A wood person needs clean, simple foods and healthy fats that are supportive to the liver:

- Dark leafy greens
- Cruciferous vegetables
- Brightly colored fruits
- Whole grains
- Legumes
- Raw nuts
- Seeds

Sour foods stimulate digestion and encourage the production of bile. Wood elemental types of people tend to enjoy sour and fermented foods:

- Citrus fruit
- Grapefruit juice
- Lemon and limeade
- Pickles
- Kimchi
- Miso
- Sauerkraut

Drink plenty of natural herbal teas that contain powerful liver cleansers:

- Chamomile
- Peppermint
- Dandelion

Clean air and pure water are especially important. Wood people need to avoid pesticides and pollutants of all sorts in order to remain healthy. Healthy nutrition will give you a clear, creative mind and high focus.

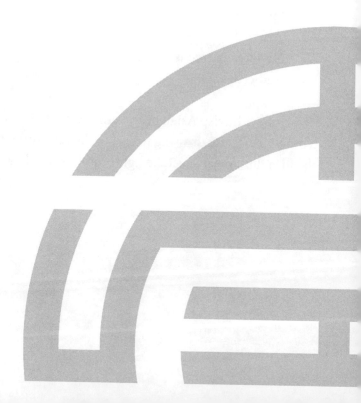

Fire Element Diet and Nutrition

Fire elemental types tend to enjoy bitter foods (dark chocolate, aperitifs, olive oil, bitter greens, coffee, black tea). In Chinese medicine, the explanation is straightforward and simple: bitter foods cool excess Fire. Fire is the hottest and most yang of all the elements, as such it tends to produce the most heat. This is why Fire elements do well with a light menu that limits alcohol and avoids excessively spicy or greasy foods. In honor of light and brightness, a Fire elements constitution benefits from cooling foods:

- Melons
- Salads
- Citrus

Because Fire elements enjoy bitterness, try salads with:

- Spinach
- Arugula
- Dandelion greens
- Radicchio

Top it off with crisp Asian pears, sunflower seeds, and a delightful lemon vinaigrette dressing to add to the refreshing taste. You get the idea. Fire meals need be light, cooling, and heart-healthy.

Earth Element Diet and Nutrition

Earth's flavor is sweet, and most Earth's enjoy sweet foods of all sorts. In order to be healthy and balanced, Earth's strengthen their energy by practicing moderation and regular dietary habits. This helps stomach energy flourish. The most fortifying foods are dense and tightly packed fruits and vegetables. Earth's should be sure to be seated and calm when they eat, in order to enjoy whatever is on their plate.

Earth energy benefits from cooked rather than raw ingredients. Food and drink are healthiest served at a warm temperature, rather than icy cold or scalding hot. In order to encourage digestion, it is important to chew food well, rather than rushing eating to get to some other activity. Grains in moderation are healing and energizing:

- Rice
- Oat
- Millet
- Yams
- Sweet potatoes

Other beneficial foods for energy are:

- Meats
- Fish
- Beans
- Nuts

This is, of course, as long as they are eaten in reasonable quantities.

Metal Element Diet and Nutrition

Pungent foods that move energy outward and upward will probably appeal to a Metal person. Pungency refers to hot and spicy foods with powerful, strong, penetrating flavors. Small amounts of them are good for the Lung Energy Network. Below are a plethora of pungent foods to try, so no single one is over-eaten.

- Garlic
- Onions
- Chili peppers
- Ginger
- Celery
- Coriander
- Fennel
- Spearmint
- Horseradish
- Fennel
- Anise
- Dill
- Radish
- Sweet peppers
- Turnips
- Mustard leaf
- Cinnamon
- Tangerine peel
- Kumquats
- Mustard seed
- Wine
- Basil
- Rosemary

- Parsley
- Coriander
- Cloves
- Cayenne

Fruits that require peeling support Metal health, particularly citrus, bananas, and mangoes. Interestingly, many of Metal elements healthiest foods are white:

- Onion
- Garlic
- Cauliflower
- Turnips
- Parsnips

During the cool and cold seasons of the year, root vegetables strengthen elemental energy:

- Potatoes
- Yams
- Turnips
- Carrots

They are easy to prepare and become deliciously caramelized when roasted in the oven.

Water Element Diet and Nutrition

The flavor of both yin and Water is salty. Salt moves energy downward and inward, stimulates appetite, and improves digestion. Salty foods include:

- Seaweed
- Celery
- Miso
- Many Asian sauces

Our kidneys require a small amount of salt in order to properly regulate water metabolism. But too much salt can damage them, not to mention increase blood pressure in susceptible persons. Black, blue, and purple foods support the kidneys and strengthens yin. Examples of foods that nourish the Water Element include:

- Blueberries
- Blackberries
- Dark grapes
- Eggplant
- Wild rice
- Blue corn
- Purple potatoes and yams

Water people will probably find that their constitution does best with cooked foods and complex carbohydrates. The sorts of dishes that are healthy for Water element people are made with:

- Whole grains
- Peas
- Squash
- Beans
- Potatoes

- Carrots
- Parsnips

Warming spices are helpful in strengthening energy. Think "cinnamon, spice, and everything nice." That is the perfect combination for Water.

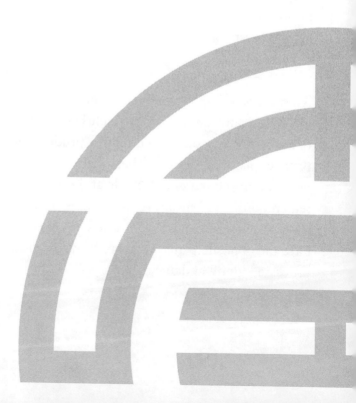

A Plant Based Diet Is the Gold Standard for Cancer Prevention

Chinese medicine has long advocated prevention, and the first line of defense against disease is your diet. The healthiest diet is one mostly based on plants and with very few animal products, such as:

- Whole grains
- Vegetables
- Fruits
- Beans
- Legumes
- Nuts
- Seeds

Large demographic studies over the last 30 years have proven the health virtues of the plant based diets of China and Japan, and yet the West continues to march to its own dietary beat. Well, not anymore.

After years of looking at the evidence between diet and cancer, the American Cancer Society published their recommendation that cancer survivors should follow "prudent diets." Specifically, prudent plant-based diets. These diets are high in fruits, vegetables, and unrefined grains, while at the same time being low in red and processed meats, refined grains, and sugars. The report states, "These diets are contrasted to 'Western' diets," which have the opposite pattern and are heavy in meats, sweets, other processed foods, and dietary fat."

It's better late than never.

Whole Soy Is Protective Against Breast Cancer

Soy is probably the most researched food in the world. Well over 100 studies have been conducted worldwide in an attempt to discover the medical benefits of this Asian staple. A majority of the studies concluded that besides soy's cholesterol lowering feature, it could actually have a breast cancer protective property. This is due to its ability to bind up estrogen-receptor sites and stop "bad" estrogen from attaching itself. In addition, several large demographic studies show cultures with high soy consumption, such as China and Japan, enjoy extremely low rates of breast cancer in women and prostate cancer in men.

We advise women to incorporate soy into their breast cancer prevention diet. But like everything we advise, we advocate balance and eating a large variety of other beans and legumes as well. Be sure to consume only whole, organic, and non-GMO soy and soy products, such as:

- Tofu
- Tempeh
- Soy milk
- Miso
- Natto

Make Sure to Beef up During Chemotherapy

There exists sound, generally agreed upon dietary principles that a high fiber, low fat, moderate protein diet is typically good for health. But in some unique circumstances, a diet rich in red meat, eggs, and other animal proteins can help. During chemotherapy, a patient's red blood cells, white blood cells, and platelets are pummeled by drugs. This causes their counts to drop dangerously. During this, an animal protein diet can increase blood production rapidly. This counteracts the need for transfusion and Epogen, a drug which stimulates bone marrow production of hemoglobin and blood cells.

When it comes to animal protein, the types from intensive factory farming leave more to be desired and often cause more harm than good. This is due to the growth hormones, antibiotics, corn, same animal meat, manure, plastics, pesticides, and other harmful things found in the feed of most conventionally farmed animals. All of this adds up to negatively affect your health. If you wouldn't want to eat it, you wouldn't want your food eating it, right?

On the other hand, grass-fed beef, organic free range livestock, and wild caught fish contain nutrients that can give a quick boost to your blood production, just when you need it the most.

Cruciferous Vegetables Activate Tumor Suppressor Genes

Cruciferous vegetables include:

- Broccoli
- Cauliflower
- Brussels sprouts
- Cabbage
- Kale
- Wasabi
- Horseradish
- Mustard
- Radish
- Watercress

They all contain isothiocyanate, a sulfur-containing compound that may help to prevent cancer. The compound does this by eliminating potential carcinogens and activating tumor suppressor genes in cells.

Studies have found isothiocyanate promotes detoxification, enhances immunity, and activates cancer inhibiting agents. It also prevents cancer of the breast, stomach, spleen, prostate, and colon. Cruciferous sprouts contain ten times higher levels of the cancer fighting chemical sulforaphane than mature vegetables. Boiling and microwaving has been shown to reduce bioavailability of sulforaphane, whereas steaming prevents the loss of the essential nutrient.

Cancer Fighting Properties of Blue and Purple Foods

The dark blue and purple pigments of fruits and vegetables contain potent antioxidants called anthocyanins. These nutrients are found in:

- Blueberries
- Blackberries
- Bilberry
- Grapes
- Red cabbage
- Red onions
- Eggplant
- Tea

Anthocyanins have been found to activate tumor suppressor genes in cancer stem cells. This triggers apoptosis (cell death) by manipulating cell signaling between cancer stem cells and tumors. Besides a handful of organic blueberries or blackberries each day, another way to get anthocyanins into your body is to make fermented sauerkraut with red cabbage and red onions. The final product is rich in both sulforaphane and anthocyanins that boost cancer stem cell-killing action.

Avocado Is a Potent Antioxidant and Anticancer Fruit

Avocado is a very popular food, especially during major league sports seasons when it is a staple along with salsa and chips. And that is a good thing, though you should be careful not to eat too many chips. Avocado contains many powerful antioxidants, including glutathione, which is nature's most important antioxidant. Glutathione prevents cellular damage caused by free radicals and is also a critical detoxifier for every cell in your body. 70% of the antioxidants in avocados are found in the seeds.

In a recent study, researchers discovered that a compound found in avocado called avocatin B was effective against acute myeloid leukemia cells. The seeds also contain flavonol, a powerful antioxidant that helps to prevent and reduce tumor growth. Besides its cancer-fighting properties, avocado is also beneficial for preventing heart disease and dementia.

Curry to the Rescue

Turmeric is a deep orange-yellow powder that is used as a spice in Indian cuisine and often found in curry dishes. It is a member of the ginger family and has been used for centuries in Chinese and Ayurvedic medicines. The active ingredient in turmeric is curcumin.

Curcumin has antioxidant, anti-inflammatory, and anti-cancer properties. It has been shown to target cancer cells by blocking elements that suppress cell death, stopping nutrients from reaching cancer cells, and halting tumor invasion and metastasis. Curcumin also promotes the production of other antioxidant compounds such as glutathione, and helps prevent damage and stress to organs.

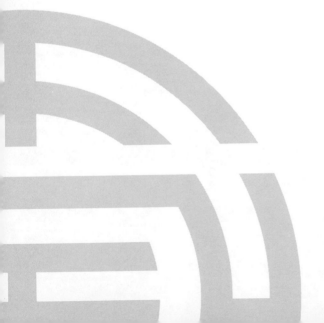

The Healing Power of Fermented Foods

Those at an increased risk of metabolic conditions and cancer usually have higher concentrations of harmful bacteria in their gut. Studies have linked an unhealthy gut with certain cancers—such as colorectal cancer, pancreatic carcinoma, and gallbladder cancer.

Fermented vegetables and beverages are excellent sources for healthy bacteria. Try adding fermented dairy-alternative products to your diet, such as:

- Almond or coconut yogurt
- Kefir with live cultures
- Sauerkraut
- Kimchi
- Tempeh
- Miso
- Kombucha
- Sourdough (with live bacteria starter)

Those Who Drink Green Tea
Have Lower Cancer Risks

Green tea has been consumed for thousands of years in China and Japan. Studies have shown that simply sipping on green tea daily can reduce the risk of breast, colon, prostate, and lung cancer. Antioxidants found in green tea have been found to prevent cancer cells from multiplying, causing inflammation, and invading new tissue. One antioxidant, epigallocatechin-3-gallate (EGCG), stops cancer cells from communicating. This prevents the formation and growth of new blood vessels in tumors. Substitute your morning cup of Joe with green tea and your body will thank you for it.

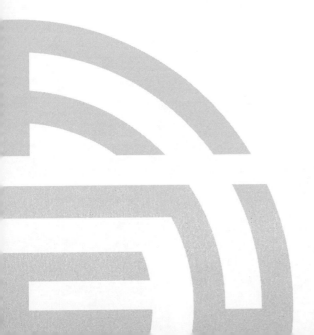

Enzymes Break Down Cancer Cell Defenses

The benefits of enzyme therapy in cancer treatment were first recognized in the early 1900s. Enzymes such as trypsin and chymotrypsin help break down the protective coating on cancer cells. This lets your immune system more effectively detect and destroy the cancer. Enzyme therapy has also helped people receiving chemotherapy. It reduces side effects such as nausea, fatigue, vomiting, and pain.

Systemic enzymes improve the immune system so that it can more effectively target cancer cells and prevent further growth. Many fruits and vegetables contain systemic enzymes. Two enzymes are papain in papaya and bromelain in pineapple, which are known for their anti-inflammatory properties.

For systemic enzymes in a supplement form, we recommend plant-based enzyme formula.

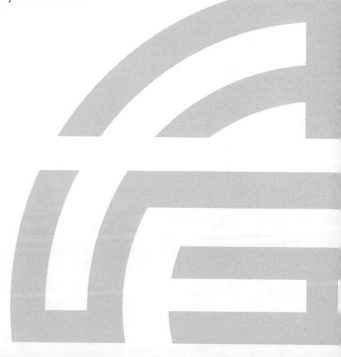

Benefits of Melatonin

Melatonin is a powerful hormone secreted by the pineal gland in your brain while you sleep. Many people don't produce enough melatonin and therefore suffer from lack of restorative sleep. A major cause of this is excessive blue light exposure at night from electronic devices, such as phones, tablets, and computers. We recommend not using any electronic devices for at least thirty minutes before bed, preferably for an hour. If you do need to use them, see if they have a night mode. Melatonin can help you enjoy better sleep. It has also been found to possess anti-cancer properties.

A review of studies published in the Journal of Pineal Research showed that melatonin lowered the risk of several types of cancer by up to 34%. It has been found to be toxic to liver, breast, prostate, lung, and brain cancers. In other words, supplemental melatonin has good potential to fight and prevent cancer.

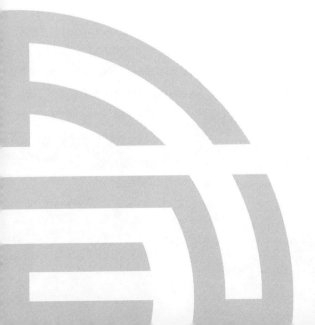

Jazz Up Your Salad and Health with Beets

The deep red color of beets is a natural wonder. It turns out both red and yellow beets have protective pigment called flavonoids, these give them their color, and antioxidant and anti-cancer properties. Studies published in Phytotherapy Research found that beets can protect against cancer by inducing cell death and shutting down genes that activate cancer cell growth and survival.

Beet's high concentration of flavonoids have strong antioxidant, anti-inflammatory, and anti-proliferative actions. It also protects the heart by helping to prevent chronic inflammation and blood vessel damage. Besides eating cooked beets, you can also add a quarter of a beet root into your vegetable juice for enhanced health.

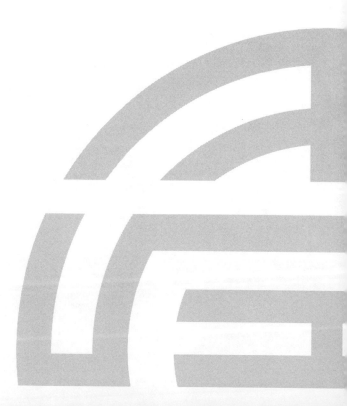

Add Sauerkraut, Pickles, or Kimchee to Your Red Meat

Studies have found that eating lots of red meat is connected to an increased risk for many cancers, especially colorectal cancer. Germans consume large amounts of red meat, and yet their rate of colorectal cancer is one of the lowest among developed countries. Their secret? Sauerkraut.

Fermented vegetables such as sauerkraut, pickles, and kimchee are a good source of healthy bacteria. They contain glucosinolates, ascorbigen, and ascorbic acid, which studies have shown decrease DNA damage and cell mutation rates in cancer patients. Sauerkraut is known to have a particularly high concentration of all these compounds. If you must eat red meat, be sure to add some sauerkraut, pickles, or kimchee to lower your cancer risks.

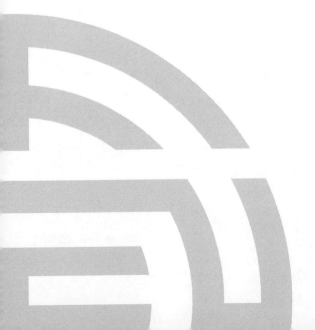

Micronutrient Testing Reveals
Precise Nutrient Deficiencies

Most people literally flush money down the toilet. Many people buy and take nutritional supplements they don't need, or even worse, buy poor quality products that don't contain contents listed on the bottle. Before you rush out and buy a bag full of nutritional supplements, we advocate performing micronutrient testing. The test will measure your nutrient levels, ranging from vitamins A-Z, amino acids, fatty acids, and antioxidants. It will also reveal specific nutrient deficiencies or excesses that require action.

Micronutrient testing can be done using either blood or urine samples. If you choose, we here at the Tao of Wellness will happily examine your test results. If you do come to us, we will first identify food sources for the deficient nutrients. After that we recommend supplementing only with high quality, bioavailable, nutritional products. Most importantly, we advocate reversing any nutritional deficiencies through your diet, as opposed to just supplements.

The Pros and Cons of a Ketogenic Diet

The ketogenic diet is low in carbohydrates and high in good fats. The calorie intake of the diet often breaks down like so:

- 75% healthy fats
- 20% proteins
- 5% or less carbohydrates

The diet's proponents claim that it can help weight loss, lower blood sugar in diabetics, and even starve cancer cells. It does this by forcing your body to burn fat instead of glucose, which in turn pushes the body into ketosis—hence the name ketogenic.

The benefit of the ketogenic diet seems to be achieved in the short term. People report weight loss, less pain and inflammation, and drops in cholesterol after only 8-10 weeks. However, the downside to the diet is that it's hard to sustain for most people. Research shows that a majority of people are unable to stay on the diet beyond three months. That may be a good thing as a diet high in fat and low in carbs may result in elevated risks for heart disease and cancer, the very disease its proponents claim it to reverse and prevent. More long term studies are needed, so for now, try it for two to three months only if you're curious, and always check with your doctor before beginning any diet regimen.

High Fiber Is Essential for Your Gut and General Health

A new study from the National Cancer Institute (NCI) found that eating fiber reduced the likelihood of death from any cause. Among the nearly 400,000 people who took part in the study, those who ate the most fiber (26-29 grams) were 22% less likely to die than those who ate the least fiber. Fiber is found in:

- Whole grains
- Beans
- Legumes
- Vegetables
- Fruits

Insoluble fiber has been found to be best for preventing colorectal cancer as it eliminates cancer-causing toxins from the colon. This type of fiber doesn't dissolve in water like those found in beans, cereal bran, and leafy greens. However, all fibers have the health benefits of lowering cholesterol, stabilizing blood sugar, and preventing cancer.

Fiber provides food for bacteria in the gut. The bacterium ferment the fiber into fatty acids, which have been found to inhibit cell breeding, encourage programmed cell death, and reduce tumor cell invasiveness. Eat at least 30 grams of fiber a day for both your gut and general health.

A Low Carbohydrate Diet Is Not Necessarily Good

A recent health trend has been to eat less carbohydrates in order to maintain health and weight. That's been good for refined carbohydrates like boxed cereals, pastries, white bread, pasta, rice, potato chips, and sugary beverages. However, it has inadvertently caused a large number of people to avoid whole grains, beans, and legumes as a result. Foods which actually promote health and do not cause weight gain.

A study was done by the US National Health and Nutrition Examination Survey. It showed that of the 24,825 participants, those with the lowest intake of carbohydrates had a 32% higher risk of all-cause death. In addition, risks of death from coronary heart disease, cerebrovascular disease, and cancer increased by 51%, 50%, and 35% respectively. This landmark study showed the importance of not completely cutting out carbohydrates from your diet. Instead, we advise that you choose complex and not refined carbohydrates for your health and longevity.

Mushrooms Are Nature's Best Immune Modulators

Mushrooms are one of the most beloved foods in Asian, Middle Eastern, and European cultures. They are prized for their nutritional content, delicate flavors, and are used in many culinary traditions. Besides being a prized food, mushrooms happen to have key bioactive compounds that are known to be immune-modulatory. This means they can enhance or suppress the immune response depending on the need. They also have been found to both reduce inflammation and protect against cancer.

Researchers from the University of Western Australia conducted a study which revealed that women who consumed at least a third of an ounce of fresh mushrooms every day were 64% less likely to develop breast cancer. Besides inhibiting cancer, they also have the ability to reduce bad estrogens which cause breast cancer. Enjoy the many varieties of delicious mushrooms, such as:

- Button
- White
- Crimini
- Shitake
- Oyster
- Portabella
- Maitake

As well as medicinal mushrooms like:

- Reishi
- Turkey tail
- Cordyceps

Complex Sugar Compounds in Yeast Activate Immune Response

Yeast cells contain a potent nutrient called beta-glucans that may help with cancer prevention. Beta-glucans are naturally occurring compounds not found in the human body. These complex sugar molecules protect the body from cancer and tumors by activating immune cells such as antibodies, natural killer cells, cytokines, T-cells, and macrophages.

Some common foods which contain beta-glucans are:
- Baker's yeast
- Oats
- Barley
- Shiitake mushrooms
- Maitake mushrooms
- Seaweed
- Algae

It has also been found to benefit heart health. In fact, beta-glucan is the key part of the cholesterol-lowering effect of oat bran. You can also take it in a supplement form.

Resveratrol: Nature's Troops Against Injury and Foreign Invaders

Resveratrol is a natural antioxidant compound produced by plants. Plants use it when they have been damaged or when under attack by bacteria or fungi. A large amount of research on resveratrol has centered on in its ability to repair and lengthen telomeres, the ends of DNAs that determine human lifespan. Resveratrol has also been found to help prevent cancer. This is because it is designed to protect cells from free radical damage and extend their lifespan. This improves the cell's ability to repair and stops them from mutating.

The cancer-protective properties of resveratrol have been shown to prevent numerous cancers, including but not limited to:
- Prostate
- Liver
- Colon
- Pancreas
- Skin

The best sources of resveratrol are the skin of fruits, such as:
- Grapes
- Blueberries
- Raspberries
- Mulberries

It may be nearly impossible to get enough of this nutrient through diet alone though, so you may want to take it as a supplement.

More Reasons to Eat More Citrus Fruits

Citrus fruits are great for disease prevention due to their high levels of essential nutrients and antioxidants. And it helps that they taste great too.

Well, now there's even more reason to eat them. A study published in the Journal of Epidemiology found that eating more citrus fruits was linked to a decreased risk of heart disease and cancer, specifically non-Hodgkin's lymphoma. Citrus fruits also contain a flavonoid called nobiletin. Nobiletin has been shown to have anti-inflammatory, cancer-fighting, and cancer cell growth suppression effects.

When eating citrus fruits such as oranges, be sure to eat the whole fruit, including the peel as that's where the most nutrients are contained. One easy way to eat the peel is to dice it up and blend into your smoothie, or dehydrate them in an oven or dehydrator and use in your cooking.

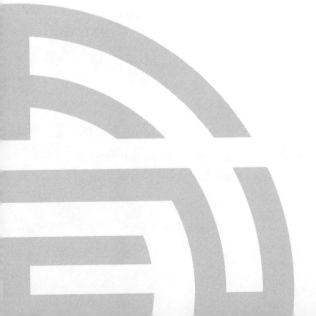

Herbs That Make Food Taste Good Are Also Good for You

Besides their pleasant aromatic tastes, many herbs contain a compound called ursolic acid. Studies have found ursolic acid to reduce tumor size and help prevent metastasis of colorectal cancer cells. This is likely by blocking the cells expression of proteins needed for their survival, proliferation, and metastasis. Studies have shown ursolic acid to help treat cancers like:

- Colon
- Breast
- Lung
- Cervix
- Prostate
- Esophagus
- Pancreas
- Skin

Some herbs used widely for cooking are:

- Basil
- Rosemary
- Oregano
- Thyme
- Peppermint
- Elderflower
- Lavender

Make these and other herbs a staple in your kitchen. By adding them to your dishes and beverages you will not only please your palate, but also improve your body's cancer fighting abilities. You may also take ursolic acid as a supplement.

Red Is Good for Your Health, so Is Lycopene

Lycopene is found in fruits and vegetables with red flesh. It is the pigment nutrient responsible for the rich red color. Lycopene's anticancer properties stem from its ability to increase cell-inhibition and programmed cell death in cancer cells. This nutrient disrupts the cancer cells' communication signals which help it to flourish, and instead increases its risk of dying. In fact, in laboratory experiments blood orange juice that contains high levels of lycopene has been shown to have potential preventative effects on leukemia cells. Other cancers that lycopene may be effective at preventing include cervix, colon, lung, and prostate cancer.

Fruits and vegetables that are high in lycopene include:
- Goji berry (wolf berry)
- Pink guava
- Papaya
- Watermelon
- Pink grapefruit
- Blood oranges
- Tomato
- Seabuckthorn
- Rose hip

Interestingly, cooking enhances the concentration of lycopene. So what are you waiting for? Make some homemade pasta sauce and salsa, bring out the watermelon on hot summer days, and snack on goji berry all year round.

Parsley, Sage, Rosemary...
Lovelier Than Meets the Eye

Flavones are present in many plants and have attracted research interest in recent years due to their bioactive properties. One flavone, apigenin, has been found to inhibit the growth of cervical carcinoma cells and stop the spread of HER2 breast cancer cells. It also exhibits reduced free radical activity and aids in the elimination of toxins from the body. As well, topical use of apigenin before UV irradiation has been found to prevent the formation of tumors in laboratory experiments.

Parsley is one of the best dietary sources of apigenin, it is also found in:

- Celery
- Chinese cabbage
- Chamomile
- Sage
- Rosemary
- Oregano

Consider juicing parsley, celery, and cabbage for concentrated amounts of apigenin in your diet.

Artichoke Is Chock-Full of Health Benefits

Artichoke contains luteolin, an anticancer flavonoid. Research has discovered that luteolin inhibits the activation of cancer cells. It does this by suppressing cancer-promoting enzymes, blocking the accumulation of carcinogens in new tissue, and protecting against the degenerative effects of cancerous activity. It also supports the elimination of toxins from inflammation, especially in the lungs, liver, and heart tissue.

Luteolin is also present in:
- Green peppers
- Radicchio
- Chicory greens

Throw radicchio in your salad, sear some shishito peppers as an appetizer, and sauté chicory greens for an anti-cancer feast.

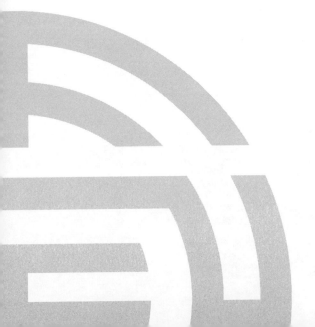

Black Pepper Is the King of Spices

As a medicinal herb, black pepper has traditionally been used in Chinese medicine to treat symptoms of cold and fever. Most recently, it has gained attention for its cancer fighting properties.

Piperine is a compound found in black pepper and responsible for its pungent flavor. Known as the "King of Spices," piperine helps reduce the incidence of cancers relating to the stomach and breast. Research has found that it has anti-inflammatory effects on Helicobacter pylori-induced gastritis, and may potentially be useful in prevention of H. pylori-associated stomach cancer.

Add black pepper to your daily diet in marinades, salad dressings, sauces, dips, and soups. Piperine can also be taken as a supplement.

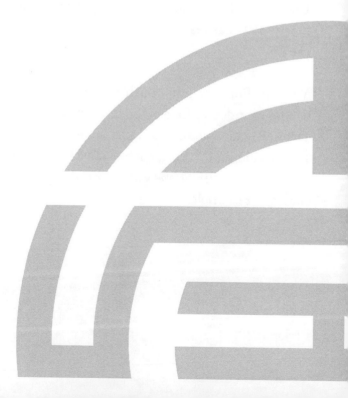

The Sunshine Vitamin in the Fight Against Cancer

Vitamin D deficiency is one of the most common factors associated with the development of cancer. Evidence of this can be found in a study of 33,000 Japanese subjects. The study found that those with a higher level of vitamin D had a 20% lower risk of cancer overall.

One of the key functions of vitamin D is its ability to reduce inflammation linked to cancer and promote the production of proteins that control cancer cells. Foods rich in vitamin D include:

- Fatty fish (salmon, tuna, mackerel)
- Beef liver
- Eggs

The sun also stimulates the body's production of vitamin D. Unfortunately, lack of daily sun exposure combined with insufficient diets has resulted in widespread vitamin D deficiency in the US.

You can find out how much vitamin D is in your system by asking your doctor for a blood test called the 25-hydroxy vitamin D test. Because vitamin D is a fat-soluble nutrient, it is important to take vitamin D3, the most bioactive kind, with a fatty meal like avocado for optimal absorption, or along with fish oil supplements, for example.

Vegetable Juicing for Antioxidants and Detoxification

Juicing has become popular and for good reason. Juicing vegetables can supply a higher amount of nutrients for absorption in comparison to eating the entire raw or cooked food on its own. Just a portion of these nutrients include glutathione, sulforaphane, flavonoids, and enzymes. Due to the massive infusion of nutrients, juicing can boost the immune system, eliminate cancer-causing toxins, and decrease the likelihood of developing cancer.

Good vegetables for juicing are:
- Kale
- Celery
- Chard
- Chinese cabbage
- Broccoli and cauliflower sprouts
- Beets
- Ginger root
- Carrots
- Blueberry
- Orange
- Parsley
- Basil
- Cucumber

You can also throw half of an apple in for taste. Start with 1/2 glass a day and over the course of a month slowly increase to 2-3 full glasses a day.

Ginger Is 10,000 Times More Potent Than Chemotherapy

Ginger root is popular in Asian cuisine and packs a punch when it comes to health benefits that span from anti-nausea to combating cancer. A study published in the Public Library of Science (PLOS) revealed a pungent, volatile oil within ginger known as 6-shogaol. This oil was found to be superior to conventional chemotherapy in targeting the root cause of breast cancer malignancy—the breast cancer stem cells. It has also been found to protect against free radical damage.

To get the full benefits of 6-shogaol, use dried ginger powder in your marinade, enjoy a cup of ginger tea, or shave it on your dishes. You can also try fermented ginger, which is commonly used with Asian dishes such as sushi and in the Korean dish kimchi.

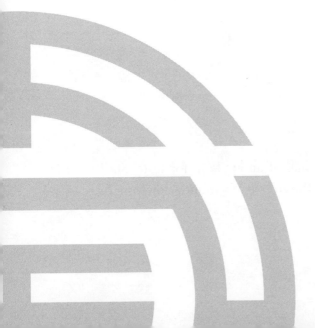

Call the Doc Instead of the Cop on the Caper

Capers are the buds of a flowering plant called Capparis. They are often used in the sauces of popular dishes, like salmon with lemon and caper sauce. This spice-bud contains many phytonutrients, antioxidants, and vitamins essential for optimum health. It also happens to be one of the best sources of the flavonoid quercetin. Quercetin has natural anti-cancer and health properties such as:

- Suppressing cancer cell proliferation.
- Reducing oxidative damage.
- Inhibiting the activity of p53 when it mutates and becomes faulty, which is associated with tumor growth.
- Stimulating the body's natural detoxification pathways.
- Helping the body's anti-inflammatory response.
- Being antihistamine.

Rich sources of quercetin include:

- Capers
- Onions
- Green and black tea
- Cacao
- Apples

You can also take it as a supplement.

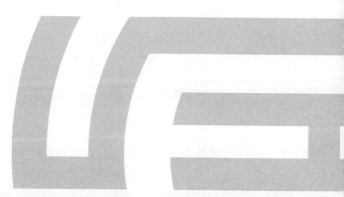

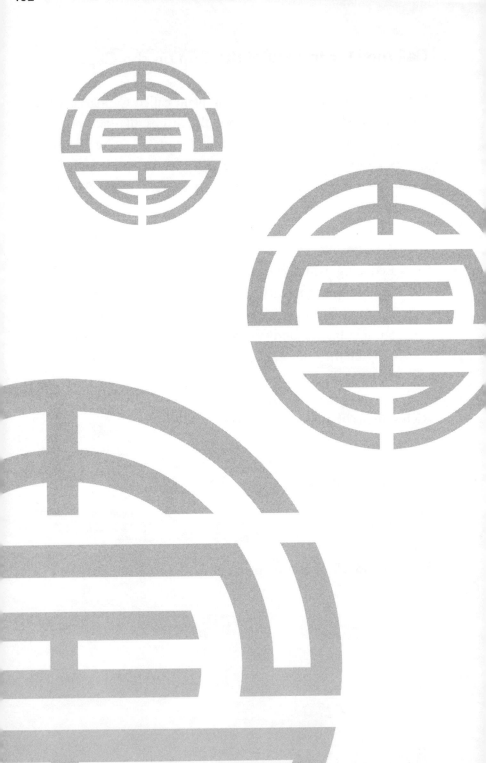

Chapter 6: What You Do — Exercise, Qi Gong, Meditation, and Sleep

The more willing you are to surrender to the energy within you, the more power can flow through you.

—*Shakti Gawain*

It has long been known that exercise on a regularly basis can help lower one's risk of disease. Now, there is increasing evidence that exercise can also lower the risk of cancer, in particular qi gong exercise.

Long before Western sciences discovered the link between the mind and body, Chinese physicians were instructing patients' of mind-body self-healing through qi gong. Qi gong works through an energy communication system within the body. By using visualization and breathing techniques, communication is restored and organ functions return to their optimal level. The benefits range from immune modulation and energy enhancement to stress reduction. And over the last 30 years, research has shown it can also help prevent cancer.

The idea behind the energy communication system governs the Chinese medical system of acupuncture. Acupuncture works through needle stimulation and activation of acupoints in the body. By doing so, the energy communication network elicits specific and intended physiological responses.   Integrating acupuncture into your health and wellness program can help you maintain healthy energy flow, and it can prevent and treat physical imbalances. Refer to Chapter 9: How You Heal for more evidence-based research on acupuncture and cancer.

Practicing qi gong can tap into the same energy communication system used by acupuncture. Studies have documented many cancer patients who have been helped by practicing qi gong and tai chi regularly. Patients who practiced these exercises have experienced a high quality of life, reduced symptoms and side effects from their cancer treatments, and an improved survival rate.

Another way to improve quality of life is meditation. Research on the benefits of meditation has shown it substantially reduces stress, inflammation, depressive symptoms, fatigue, and insomnia. As well, a majority of people who use daily meditation report positive feelings of peace and meaning. I cringe every time I hear the refrain, "I'll sleep more when I'm dead." America is a sleep deprived nation and that has huge implications on one's health. Sleep deprivation leads to an elevated risk of heart disease, obesity, and cancer.

This chapter will discuss the benefits of mind-body exercises and meditation, as well as how to implement sleep training into your life in order to get restorative sleep. You will also find Qi Gong Meditation for Cancer Support outlined in the latter half of this chapter so that you can practice at home for the maximum boost in health and wellness.

Being Physically Active
Lowers the Risk of Cancer Recurrence

For most people, a sedentary lifestyle carries the same risk of heart disease and cancer as smoking a pack of cigarettes a day. For instance, studies of 35,522 cancer survivors showed that physical activity after a cancer diagnosis was connected with 32-40% lower risk of cancer recurrence and 38% lower mortality rate.

Physical activity simply means moving throughout the day and not staying still. There's no wrong way of being active. Walking, gardening, pushing a baby stroller, climbing the stairs, playing soccer, dancing, and more all count.

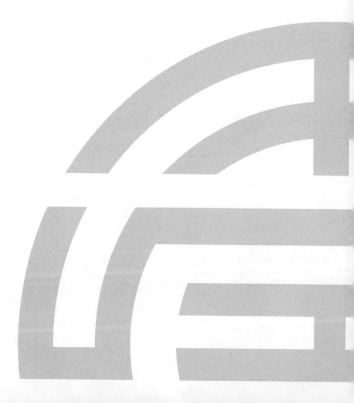

Qi is Energy, Life Force, and Represents Essential Vitality

To gain mastery over our lives and achieve optimal health, it is necessary to have a basic understanding of the nature of energy. Qi, also known as vital energy or life force, is the subtle breath of life that permeates and vitalizes the universe. It is formless energy that envelops us and fills us. Just as a fish is unaware of the fact that it lives in water, we are unaware of the inexhaustible sea of energy that supports our lives.

The sun is an example of this energy. It provides fuel for plant life, it activates biological clocks in humans and other organisms, and its energy can even be converted into electricity for use in our homes and offices. But most of the energy around us is imperceptible, that's why we call it subtle energy.

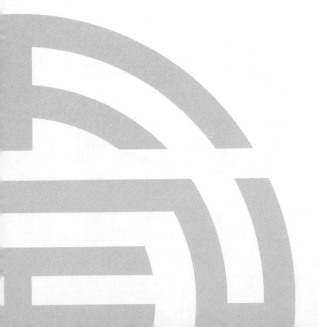

Qi Activates and Sustains All Life

Subtle energy gives birth to life. Everything that exists is an expression or projection of that energy in varying states. For a more in-depth description, here is a quote from my book, Secrets of Self-Healing:

When qi gathers, it is called matter. When qi diffuses, it is called space. When qi animates form it is called life. When qi separates and withdraws from form, it is called death. When qi flows, there is health. When qi is blocked, there is sickness and disease. Qi embraces all things, circulates through them, and sustains them. The planets depend on it for their light and motion, weather is formed by it, and seasons are caused by it. Qi activates and sustains all life.

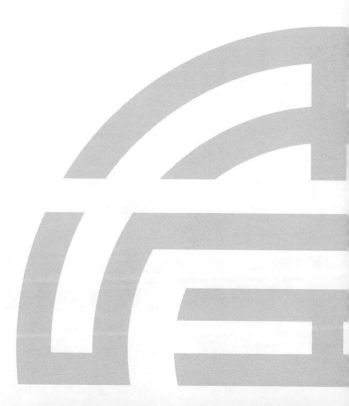

Measuring Qi

Qi is informational, it carries a specific signal or message. It is similar to how voices or data are carried by electrical currents, by bursts of light through fiber-optic cables, and by radiofrequency through cellular or Wi-Fi signals. These are all energy.

Our bodies are absorptive, reflective, and generative of informational energy fields. We can now record and measure that energy. For instance, an electroencephalogram (EEG) records the electrical signals from brain waves. Studies show that when a medical qi gong practitioner is emitting energy towards a subject, there is a shift of EEG brain wave patterns to the alpha state (the healing and resting state) in the subject. Recent studies have also shown that meditative states cause similar changes in the brain waves.

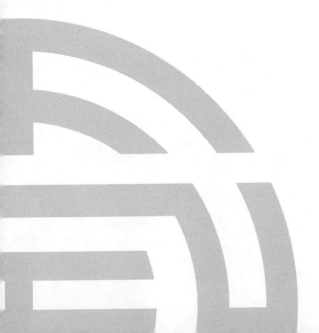

Qi Gong Improves Energy

Qi gong is a mind-body exercise from traditional Chinese medicine. It is used to prevent disease and augment medical treatments in order to improve health and energy levels through regular practice. A study published in the Journal of Clinical Oncology found that practicing medical qi gong at the same time as ongoing treatment can reduce fatigue and improve quality of life in cancer patients. This study supports the use of medical qi gong as an adjunct for cancer patients.

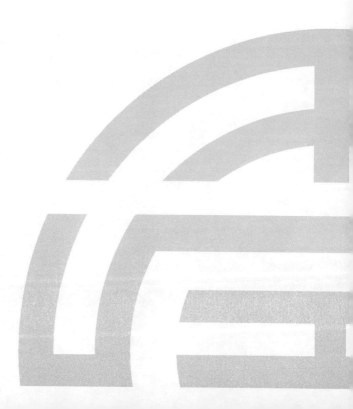

Qi Gong Improves Quality of Life

Studies from the journals Integrative Cancer Therapies, Annals of Behavioral Medicine, Clinical Journal of Oncology Nursing, as well as studies from multiple institutions all came to the same conclusion: Qi gong improves quality of life. Those who practiced it had reductions in fatigue, depression, inflammation, and sleep disturbances. Moreover, it helped raise patients moods.

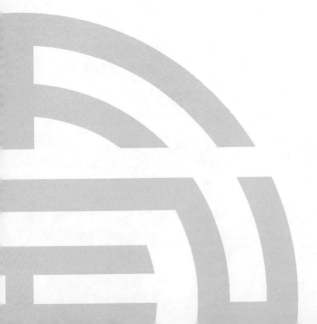

Mindfulness Meditation
Reduces Stress and Enhances Wellbeing

Research has shown that mindfulness meditation helps reduce the psychological and physical suffering of people living with cancer. These benefits include reductions in stress, as well as enhanced coping and well-being. Clinicians and researchers are excited to include mindfulness meditation in cancer care.

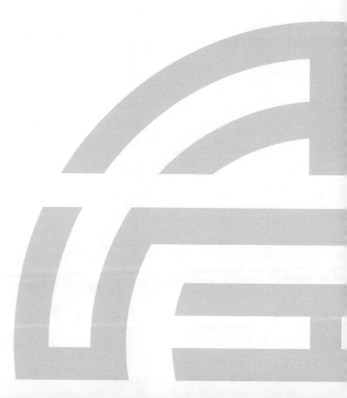

Qi Gong Improves
Neuropathy and Sexual Function

A study published in the International Journal of Physical Medicine and Rehabilitation demonstrated that qi gong has the potential to relieve nerve damage caused by cancer treatments. Woman with metastatic breast cancer who practiced qi gong and meditation had improvements in quality of life, fatigue, stress, and sexual functions.

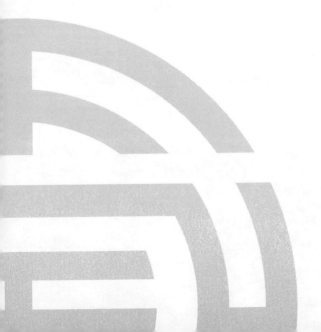

Meditation Reduces Inflammation

A study in the journal Cancer evaluated the effectiveness of mindfulness meditation for premenopausal breast cancer survivors. The findings showed a considerable decrease in stress and a reduction in inflammation.

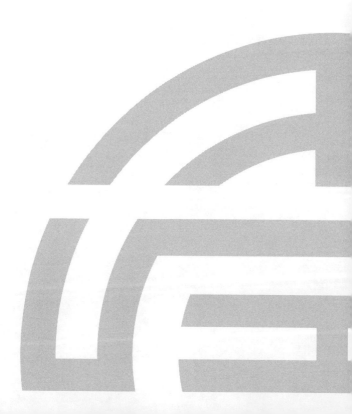

Mindfulness-based Therapies Significantly Reduced Anxiety

In a review of 1,403 participants on the effects of mindfulness-based therapies the results were overwhelmingly positive. The studies showed that adult cancer patients and survivors had "significantly reduced symptoms of anxiety and depression from pre- to post treatment." This evidence supports including mindfulness based therapies for cancer patients and survivors to help reduce anxiety and depression.

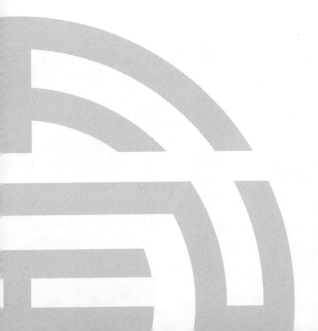

Mindfulness-based Stress Reduction Improved Cognitive Function

Cognitive impairment is a common, fatigue related symptom caused by cancer. Researchers ran a study on mindfulness-based stress reduction (MBSR) and its effects on cancer-related cognitive impairment. The study presents evidence that suggests MBSR may help the cognitive functions of cancer survivors with fatigue.

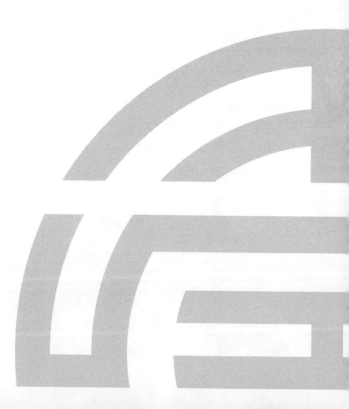

Guided Imagery and Progressive Muscle Relaxation Leads to Reduced Pain and Fatigue

A study of patients receiving chemotherapy showed that Guided Imagery (GI) and Progressive Muscle Relaxation (PMR) decreased side effects, such as:

- Fatigue
- Pain
- Nausea
- Vomiting
- Retching

Additionally, it increased quality of life. The study demonstrated the importance of using GI and PMR in the management of chemotherapy induced side effects.

Refer to later pages of this chapter on Stress Release Meditation with guided imagery.

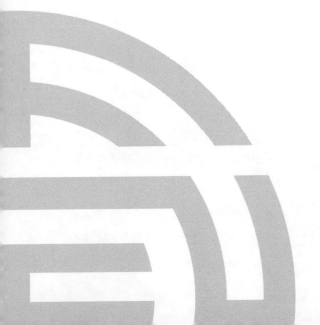

Relaxation Techniques Have a Positive Effect on Stress

A study was conducted with a group of breast cancer patients from Taiwan who were receiving both relaxation techniques and guided imagery before chemotherapy. The patients were also given instructions to practice for 20 minutes daily for 7 days after chemotherapy. At the end of the study, those who practiced had strong reductions in:

- Insomnia
- Pain
- Anxiety
- Stress
- Depression

The study concluded that incorporating relaxation techniques with guided imagery has a "positive effect on mediating anxiety and depression in breast cancer patients."

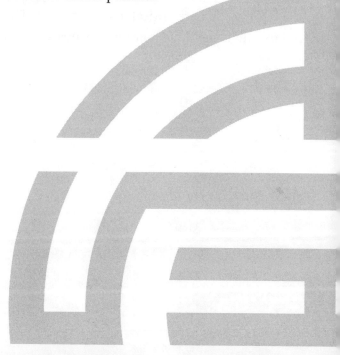

Get a Daily Dose of Sun for Increased Health and Healing

The ancient Greeks recognized the health benefits of sunlight and called it heliotherapy. Studies show that healthy amounts of exposure to sunlight can increase production of vitamin D, which is essential for immune function and cancer prevention. It also can improve your mood and help create optimism.

Due to skin cancer scares, a majority of people in northern hemisphere developed countries have shunned direct sun exposure. As a result, they are missing out on one of nature's wonder cures.

The sun provides a tremendous benefit for those looking to prevent or slow the growth of cancer. Fair skinned individuals should try getting 15-20 minutes of high quality sun exposure a day, while darker skinned individuals should aim for up 45 minutes. Be sure not to use sunscreen so you are able to absorb the UV rays that are critical to good health. The best time to go out for sun is the three hours after sunrise and before sunset.

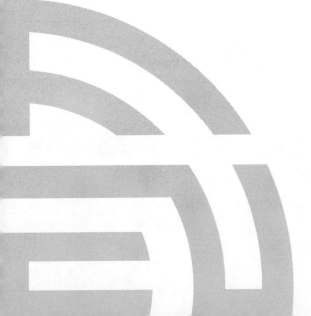

A Good Night Sleep is Critical
for a Healthy Immune System

Do you toss and turn all night long only to dream of getting a good night's rest? Chronic sleep deprivation affects almost two out of every three Americans and can increase your risk of disease and compromise your immune system.

During sleep you cycle through five phases. Each phase helps your body undergo important organ repair and regeneration. During the third and fourth phases, hormones are released and tissue repair begins. In order to receive the full benefits of rest and reach each phase, sleep should be uninterrupted. The average adult needs 7 to 9 hours of sleep per night, while older adults, past the age of 65, may only need 7 to 8 hours of sleep per night on average. Beyond the number of hours, quality is also important. Sleep apnea and other disorders can compromise sleep quality. Seek testing and help with a certified sleep specialist if you suspect sleep apnea. Otherwise, read on to discover some pillow-friendly secrets to help you slip into a deeper and more restful slumber.

Sleep Training to the Rescue

If you have children you probably understand the need for sleep training them. It's usually a variation on a routine like dinner, bath, story time, and lights out. As adults we lose this training by becoming distracted by online devices, TV programs, and anxiety and worries about the next day. But that can be avoided by training yourself to have a good night's sleep, similar to the training that your parents used on you. Here are simple steps to follow in order to enjoy a good, restorative sleep.

1. Set an alarm for one hour before bedtime.
2. Go around the house and dim all the lights. Also be sure to put away blue-light emitting devices such as TVs, computers, tablets, and smartphones. The blue-light they emit disturbs your circadian rhythm. If you must use these devices, wear blue light blocking glasses.
3. Start winding down by doing a brain dump. Empty your thoughts onto a journal, but do not analyze, plan, or problem solve.
4. Take a hot bath with Epsom salt to relax your muscles.
5. Get into bed, meditate, and actively let go of any remaining thoughts, this will hasten your descent into your sleep cycle.

Practice this routine nightly to ensure consistent quality of sleep.

Tao of Wellness' Qi Gong Meditation for Cancer Support

The founders at Tao of Wellness have developed a simple Qi Gong Meditation program for our patients based on over 30 years of research and clinical experience. It consists of four parts:
- Stress Release Meditation
- Foundation Qi Gong
- Five Elements Clearing & Harmonizing Qi Gong
- Qi Gong for Detoxification

In the following pages you will find instructions on how to practice the Qi Gong for Cancer Support. (You may also want to log on to taoofwellness.com to download an instructional video to your device.)

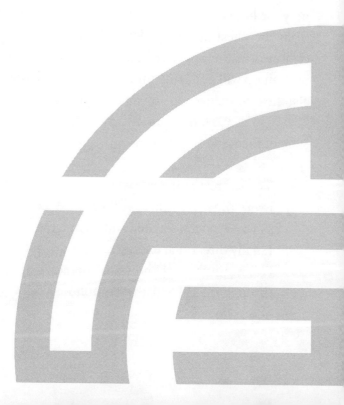

Part I: Stress Release Meditation

The purpose of this breathing meditation is to move energy down and away from your head to release stress or built-up tension.

Start by either standing, sitting, or lying down.

- It is preferable to sit comfortably with both legs and thighs forming a 90-degree angle and your feet approximately shoulder width apart.
- The lying down position is the preferred position for those who have a hard time sitting or standing.

In the beginning, breathe naturally. After practicing a few times, try to breathe with your abdomen only. Do this by breathing from the bottom up. Relax, close your eyes for three minutes, and breathe. Like a baby, breathe from low in your abdomen, pulling up your lungs from the bottom. Many people breathe primarily from the chest and shoulders, which only worsens feelings of tightness in the upper section of the torso. Breathing from the bottom up will gradually undo this pattern of breathing, and can also help to relieve tension and support a more natural posture. Try to be relaxed, tranquil, and peaceful. Your mind will be in a state of focused relaxation.

1. Slowly breathe in and out.
2. Every time you exhale say the word "calm" in your mind as you visualize an area and its muscles relax.
3. Finally direct that energy further down the pathway. Follow these steps and visualize moving the qi energy through the three pathways outlined below to complete one cycle.

Follow the pathways in order of 1, 2, and 3 to complete one cycle. After the three pathways concentrate quietly and peacefully on the "Dan Tien" for three minutes. The Dan Tien is the energy center in your abdomen, below the belly button. Afterwards, repeat 2 more cycles or as many as it takes for you to become free from stress and tension.

The Three Pathways of Stress Release with Guided Imagery

During this practice remember to slowly breathe in and out. Every time you exhale say the word "calm" in your mind as you visualize an area and its muscles relaxing. Then direct the energy further down the pathway.

Pathway 1:

Start on both sides of the head, then move down both sides in this order:

1. Neck
2. Shoulders
3. Upper arms
4. Elbows
5. Forearms
6. Wrists
7. Hands
8. Fingers

At the end, concentrate at the tip of both middle fingers for about 1 minute.

If you are suffering from numbness or tingling in your fingertips, visualize the toxins that caused that neuropathy evaporating as black smoke from your fingertips.

Pathway 2:

Start on the face, then move down the front of your body in this order:

1. Throat
2. Chest
3. Abdomen
4. Front of the thighs
5. Knees
6. Legs
7. Top of the feet
8. Toes

At the end, concentrate on the tips of both big toes for about 1 minute. Again, if you are suffering from numbness or tingling in your toes, visualize the toxins of that neuropathy evaporating as black smoke from the tips of your toes

Pathway 3:

Start on the back of the head, then move down the backside in this order:

1. Neck
2. Shoulders
3. Upper back
4. Lower back
5. Back of the thighs

6. Back of the knees
7. Calves
8. Heels
9. Bottom of the feet

At the end, concentrate at the sole of the feet for about 3 minutes.

Returning the Energy Back to the Energy Center

After completing all three pathways, concentrate and gather the energy back to the Dan Tien (the energy center in the lower abdomen).

1. Place your left palm directly on the lower abdomen, and your right hand will cup over the left.
2. Move the hands together in a circular, clockwise motion 36 times. Start with small circles and build to larger ones.
3. Then repeat 36 more times in the reverse direction.
4. When you're finished circling, rub both palms together to generate heat
5. Then cup your hands over your eyes and feel the heat permeate them.
6. Now you can slowly open your eyes, rise, and return to normal activity.

Part 2: Foundation Qi Gong

Foundation Qi Gong exercises are used to loosen and open up the various joints of the body. This allows blood, qi, and body fluids to pass through the entire body with ease. When practiced regularly you will experience more graceful movements, minimized muscle and joint strain, and increased strength and energy. Moreover, physical and emotional stressors are released during the short routines outlined in the following pages.
(You may also want to log into taoofwellness.com to download an instructional video.)

Tapping

Before we get started, it is important to mention what tapping is in qi gong. It uses the inner side of your fist, and mainly your thumb and index finger should connect. It is not a hard motion. Just a gentle, friendly tap to get the energy moving.

Tapping the Trunk to Awaken Qi Life Force

1. Place your feet shoulder width apart with your arms hanging loose at your sides.
2. Turn your pelvis while shifting your weight back and forth. Imagine you are turning to look behind you, just without moving your legs or feet. This should create momentum enough for your arms to swing in front and behind you.
   - Your weight should mostly be on the left leg while turning the pelvis to the left, and then shifted to the opposite leg as your position changes.

3. While your arms are swinging, use loose fists to alternately tap the lower abdomen below the navel and at a similar height on the back. Repeat this movement several times.

4. Continue this turning and tapping while raising where your fists land, moving from the lower abdomen up to the shoulders, and mirroring this tapping by moving your fists up your back as well. Then tap back down the same path, ending where you started on the lower abdomen and back.

Tapping the Arms to Move Qi to the Hands

1. With your feet shoulder width apart, extend your left arm forward at shoulder height.

2. Making a loose fist with your right hand. Lightly tap your trunk, starting just beneath the navel, and move upward along your left side to beneath your left armpit.

3. Tap up to your left shoulder and then to the neck, move back down your shoulder and down the inside of your left arm to the palm.

4. Then tap up the outside of your left arm, back up to the shoulder and neck.

5. When finished, gently shake out your left arm.

6. Repeat this sequence on your right side while tapping with your left fist.

Tapping the Back and Legs to Move Qi to the Feet

1. Start by rubbing your palms in a circular motion over your lower back and kidney area a few times. The circle should move up the spine, then downwards alongside the spine.
2. With loose fists, tap over your lower back in a similar circular pattern several times.
3. Next, place your feet wide apart with your legs straight.
4. Bend at the waist, and using the palm side of your fists, tap down the outside of the buttocks, thighs, legs, and ankles.
5. Tap up the inner ankles, legs, and thighs, straightening your body as you go.
6. Bring your feet back to shoulder width apart.
7. Tap the area that connects the thighs to the pelvis several times and, with each tap, alternate between slightly bent and straightened knees.

Swing the Arms and Jump for Activation of the Cardiovascular

1. Place your feet shoulder width apart.
2. Gently swing your arms downward in front of your body and behind to the back, letting the swing take your arms upward.
3. Reverse the swing from the back to the front.
4. Repeat this several times, inhaling as your arms move backward and exhaling as they come forward.
5. Allow a natural resistance to inform you how far to swing them in either direction.

6. Enhance the swing by bending your knees as your arms swing down past the front of your body. As your arms reach up in the back, lift your heels.

7. After several more swings, jump up as your arms move back and up. You should feel the backward/upward movement of your arms naturally carries you into a jump at the end of the swing. Jump several times, going higher with each swing.

8. Then progressively jump smaller until you stop jumping, slowing the back and forth of the arm swing until you're standing naturally still.

This practice has been shown to improve cardiovascular capacity.

Joint Rotations to Open and Lubricate Joints

Once vital energy, blood circulation, and the lymphatic system are awakened by tapping your trunk and extremities, we need to be sure that the qi energy isn't obstructed at the joints. Within the foundation qi gong practice are movements that circle the joints and open up the movement of fluids that nourish and restore joint functions. These joint rotations should be done gently and slowly, without any strain whatso ever.

With consistent practice you will naturally experience an increase in your range of motion.

Neck Rotation

1. Place your heels together and face your feet forward.
2. Place your left hand on the lower abdomen, with the right hand on top of the left.
3. Gently tilt your torso to the left side, allowing your head to lean to the left, then the back, right, and front. Allow gravity to do the work in moving your head.
4. Repeat three times in each direction, inhaling as the head goes back and exhaling as it comes forward again.
5. During this whole body movement, allow your head to follow the gravitational pull.

Hip and Waist Rotation

1. Start with your feet wide apart (double the width of your shoulders) and legs straight.
2. Place your hands on the sides of your waist and bend forward.
3. Keeping your hands in place, turn from the waist and bring your upper body to the left, circling up to standing with a slight back bend, down to the right side, before bending forward again. Inhale when circling to the back, exhale when circling to the front.
4. Repeat three times in both directions.

Knee Rotation

1. With your feet together, bend at the waist and rest your hands on your knees. Gently rub them to warm them up.

2. Keeping your palms centered on the upper ridge of the kneecaps, bend your knees to make a circle, pushing toward your left side, circling them around in front, then to the right side, and finally straightening back up.
3. Repeat three times in both directions.
4. Next, keeping your knees together, bend them forward and then separate to each side, circling back to center as you straighten your legs. Repeat three times.
5. Reverse the direction of the circles and repeat three more times.
6. Exhale when your knees bend down, inhale when straightening the legs.

Ankle Rotation

1. Lift your left foot and rotate it at the ankle three times in both directions.
2. Point and extend the foot, then shake the ankle and the entire leg to loosen the joints.
3. Repeat for your other foot. Your breathing should be deep and natural.

Shoulder rotation

1. Lift your left shoulder and roll it backward, down, forward, and up, making sure to keep your arms relaxed.
2. Repeat three times in each direction.
3. Repeat on your right shoulder.
4. Inhale while circling up and exhale while circling down.

1. Extend both arms out perpendicular to your body.
2. Rotate your arms from the shoulder joints by turning your hands in a circle as far in one direction as you can and then repeat in the other direction.
3. Do this three times and feel the upper arm turning inside the shoulder joint on each side.

Wrist Rotation

1. Clasp your hands together with your fingers interlaced.
2. Leading with the thumbs, trace a horizontal figure 8 in front of your body with your hands, making sure to maximize the range of motion with your wrists.
3. You can start with a small figure 8 and gradually make it larger with each revolution, before reversing the motion to lead with the pinkies, and making the figure 8 move ments smaller once again.
4. Breathe naturally and deeply.

Shaking Down the Tree

1. Start with your feet shoulder width apart, your spine straight, and your arms hanging loosely by your sides.
2. Gently bounce your whole body, focusing on your center of gravity around the pelvis area.
3. The bouncing should start at the balls of your feet and all the joints should be involved in the motion. While most of the movement will come from bending your knees, this motion should cause a gentle vibration to move the energy to all parts of your body.

4. Sometimes you will bounce vigorously and other times more gently. Follow what your body needs in the moment.

5. This bouncing movement can be performed on its own for a few seconds or up to several minutes at a time when a simple body-wide stimulation and relaxation is desired.

6. When completed, take a moment to feel the sensations moving through your body.

Vibrating the body in this way has been repeatedly shown to promote bone strength. And when bones are strong, the tissues and joints attached to them are strong as well.

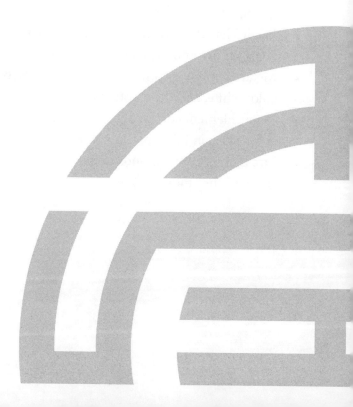

Part 3: Five Elements Clearing & Harmonizing Qi Gong

This qi gong exercise is designed to clear obstructions of qi energy and sooth stagnant emotions.

It recognizes emotional stagnation as a source of stress that can lead to physical ailments, such as cancer. Often, these stresses are trapped in each of the five Elements and their respective organ networks. Using the power of visualization, color, and breath you will learn to clear these emotional traumas and harmonize your body, mind, and spirit to attain peace, health, and joy. Below, you will find the Five Elements and their respective systems. (You may also want to log into taoofwellness.com to download an instructional video to your device.)

- Wood Element corresponds to the Liver Network, color green, and the emotion of anger.
- Earth Element corresponds to the Stomach Network, the color yellow, and the emotion of worry.
- Metal Element corresponds to the Lung Network, the color white, and the emotion of grief.
- Water Element corresponds to the Kidney Network, the color blue, and the emotion of fear.
- Fire Element corresponds to the Heart Network, the color red, and the emotion of hurt.

How to Practice the Five Elements Clearing & Harmonizing Qi Gong

1. Begin this practice by visualizing your qi energy in the Dan Tian energy center, in your lower abdomen.
2. From there move it up the spine and down your arms to your hands.
3. Designating your right hand as the emitter and left as the receiver you will move a particular color light energy from your right emitter hand into the corresponding organ network. This will clear the respective emotional stagnation and transform the negative emotion into red color light.
4. From there move it to your heart
5. Then to the left receiver hand, held about a foot from our heart.
6. Shake out the left hand and then continue onto the next Element.

Wood Element Harmonizing Qi Gong

1. Put your right hand over your liver, located in the right rib area under your breast.
2. Visualize green light emitted from your right hand clearing anger, depression, and frustration from your liver network.
3. Move the light to the heart where it is transformed by the power of love, compassion, and forgiveness into red light and received by your left hand.
4. Shake out the left hand and let go of any remaining negative attachment.

Earth Element Harmonizing Qi Gong

1. Put your right hand over your stomach in the center of your upper abdomen.
2. Visualize yellow light emitted from your right hand clearing worry, anxiety, and rumination from your stomach network.
3. Move the light to the heart where it is transformed by the power of love, compassion, and forgiveness into red light and received by your left hand.
4. Shake out the left hand and let go of any remaining negative attachment.

Metal Element Harmonizing Qi Gong

1. Put your right hand over your right chest area.
2. Visualize white light emitted from your right hand clearing grief, loneliness, and loss from your lung network.
3. Move the light to the heart where it is transformed by the power of love, compassion, and forgiveness into red light and received by your left hand.
4. Shake out the left hand and let go of any remaining negative attachment.

Water Element Harmonizing Qi Gong

1. Put your right hand over your kidney in the lower right area of your back.
2. Visualize blue light emitted from your right hand clearing fear, fright, and insecurity from your kidney network.
3. Move the light to the heart where it is transformed by the power of love, compassion, and forgiveness into red light and received by your left hand.
4. Shake out the left hand and let go of any remaining negative attachment.

Fire Element Harmonizing Qi Gong

1. Put your right hand over your heart in the left chest area.
2. Visualize red light emitted from your right hand clearing hurt, disappointment, and broken-heartedness from your heart network.
3. Then focus on the heart, where it is transformed by the power of love into red light and received by your left hand.
4. Shake out the left hand and let go of any remaining negative attachment.

Part 4: Qi Gong for Detoxification

1. Take a deep breath.
2. Visualize energy flowing from your Dan Tien in your lower abdomen down to the perineum and back up the spine to the base of your neck.
3. Bring your arms up to your sides, palms up, parallel with the floor.
4. Next bring your hands forward in front of chest and crisscross them in front of the upper body.
5. Move the tips of your middle fingers on both hands to make contact with at the high point of your upper shoulders, where you may feel a lot of tension knots.
6. Now exhale.
7. Allow the energy to move from your spine through your arms and out the middle fingers into both upper shoulders.
8. Guide your energy down through your whole body, through both legs and out the bottom of your feet. Think of it as if you're hooked up to a shower and rinsing the inside of your body out, getting rid of impurities as the cleansing energy drains down the legs and out the bottom of your feet.

Continue to repeat this breathing pattern along with the visualization of energy movement. Do this continuously for at least five minutes. (You may also want to log into taoofwellness.com to download an instructional video to your device.)

Chapter 7: Who You Are — Faith, Beliefs, and Resilience

Over-indulgence of the five emotions damages the Qi (energy), which protects and nourishes the five organs systems. When the Qi is injured, the body is vulnerable to attacks by the vicious pathogens, yin and yang become out of balance, organs malnourished, disease and even death may ensue soon thereafter.

—Yellow Emperor's Classic of Medicine

An effective immune system maintains a balance that neither overreacts nor underreacts. In the case of cancer, an effective immune system identifies the renegade cells at the earliest stage of imbalance. It then seeks to rebalance by either eliminating the cancer cell at its infancy or inhibiting its further progression. However, sometimes it fails to catch the renegade cells and allows them to grow into tumors. The process of destroying cancer and invading pathogens, like a virus or bacteria, involves inflammation. Normally, once the healing is complete, the immune system turns off the inflammation and health is restored. But in abnormal situations the inflammation persists and becomes destructive, potentially contributing to the damage of cellular DNAs and leading to cancerous changes.

So why does one's immune system succeed most of the time but fall short sometimes? What makes your immune system vulnerable and dysfunctional? You cannot expect a healthy immune function without understanding the main cause of its breakdown in the modern age: stress, the Achilles heel of immunity. Stress' negative impact on health has long been recognized by Chinese medicine, even before the discovery of the fight or flight response in modern science. Now, modern research has confirmed stress' negative influence on health and wellbeing.

In the Yellow Emperor's Classic of Medicine, considered to be the oldest book on medicine in the world, stress' harm to health and longevity was recognized in the following passage: "Over-indulgence of the five emotions damages the qi (energy), which protects and nourishes the five organs systems. When the qi is injured, the body is vulnerable to attacks by the vicious pathogens, yin and yang become out of balance, organs malnourished, disease and even death may ensue soon thereafter."

In 1980, psychologist Claus Bahnson found that patients with cancer were more likely to have suffered severe personal loss at an early age, and be depressed with strong, persistent feelings of helplessness and hopelessness. It has been concluded that people with a particular personality are much more prone to developing cancers. This personality appears in those who experience prolonged stress and tend to deny and repress their own feelings.

In the East, 5,000 years ago, Chinese medicine mapped out five distinct personalities called Five Elements Personalities. Each Element exhibiting positive and negative qualities and traits, as well as health strengths and vulnerabilities, which includes certain diseases like cancer. Research suggests that personality creates stress, which in turn deteriorates health. Some cancer survivors concur and report that they believe their personality does increase the stress they feel compared to their peers with different personalities. By understanding who you are, your personality tendencies and quirks, you can work on accentuating your strengths and improving your weaknesses. Thus, you become more capable of coping with changes that often cause stress.

In the West, cardiologists Meyer Friedman and RH Rosenman coined the terms Type A, Type B, and Type C personalities. A Type A is someone who exhibits intense emotions outwardly, such as anger, frustration, and impatience. In contrast, a Type B personality is more laid back, relaxed, and tolerant. Type C personality is prone to have difficulty expressing their feelings and have a tendency to suppress or repress emotions they consider negative, inappropriate, or uncomfortable. Research shows Type C's have a higher lifetime risk of developing cancer.

Your perception, beliefs, and faith loom large in how you ultimately cope with life situations that may cause stress. Obviously, what may be traumatic to one person may not have any effect on another. Your emotional reaction is very much based on your vantage point of a given situation, your judgement of the various pieces based on your beliefs, and your outlook on how it may resolve and conspire to create either a negative or positive emotional reaction in you. We have witnessed firsthand how our patients have used cancer as an opportunity for change. In other words, these cancer survivors often seized on it to shift course in their own lives, for the better.

Many studies in recent years have solidified our understanding of the impact of emotional stress on the body, in particular the immune and endocrine systems. Psychoneuroimmunology and neuroendocrinology are the two new fields to have emerged from these studies on the connection between the mind and emotions in three important systems, namely:

- The autonomic nervous system
- The immune system
- The endocrine system

This chapter will introduce you to techniques for stress management, ranging from meditation, creative visualization, and prayer, to building a community of support and cultivating faith and resiliency. These techniques will help reverse the destructive impact of stress and help increase your health and wellbeing, which leads to lowered risks for all diseases.

It's Time We Deal with the Big "C" with Candor, Empathy, and Knowledge

The big "C" is a scary and taboo subject. Despite the sobering number of cases, many people are afraid to discuss cancer in our culture. It's awkward socially. For example, what do you say to someone who was just diagnosed or is in the middle of treatment for cancer? Perhaps you're fearful of saying anything that might make this person feel bad. Do you offer advice or sympathy? Do you acknowledge their fear? Or do you simply clam up and say nothing? It's time we stop skirting around the subject and deal directly with the disease and the people who are living with it. And to do so with candor, empathy, and knowledge. Avoidance of the topic robs us of the opportunity to consider steps that can be taken to prevent cancer in the majority of people; while discussion helps patients better manage their condition and perhaps even experience improved quality of life.

Cancer Is a Danger but Also an Opportunity for Change

Once patients recover from the initial shock of a cancer diagnosis, we begin to explore the Chinese concept of danger with them. In Chinese, danger is called wei ji. It is comprised of the two characters: wei, danger, and ji, opportunity. It's normal to feel frightened, paralyzed, and defeated when faced with a cancer diagnosis. However, ask yourself, what's the meaning, message, and opportunity in this? In other words, cancer begs the question, "What is not working for you and how would you like to change it?"

If you want to overcome cancer and prevent its occurrence or recurrence you must change the patterns in your life that lead to the disease in the first place. Maybe it's the toxic environment, hurtful relationships, meaningless work, or unfulfilled dreams in your life. If you are not getting what you want out of your life, ask for it. Cancer is strangely empowering because it gives someone the power to make the changes that they otherwise would not be compelled to. Whatever it may be, you have nothing to lose except not seizing the opportunity for change to make your life better, happier, and healthier.

Cancer Had Awakened a Dormant Dream

Years ago, a young woman showed up in my office with stage four melanoma that had metastasized to her lungs and liver. Her oncologist had given her a very poor prognosis and three to six months to live. She was devastated and distraught and cried through our entire consultation appointment. After her tears had dried, I asked her if there was a dream that she had that remained unfulfilled to which she replied, "I always dreamt of swimming with wild dolphins in the ocean since I was a little girl." Well, as life would have it, I had a friend return from Hawaii a week prior and hand me a business card with the words "Dolphin Quest Guide" on it.

I handed her the card and a short time later she flew to Hawaii and went swimming with the dolphins in Captain Cook's Bay. She stayed for one month and was in the ocean every day. Later, she returned to Hawaii and apprenticed with the guide and eventually became one herself. A year later, I went to Hawaii to experience the same magic she had experienced with the dolphins. It was an experience that I will never forget. The best part of this story is that her cancer went into remission without treatment and she lived for fifteen years after her initial diagnosis. This was far longer than her initial prognosis. In her own words, "Cancer had awakened a dormant dream and my life was better because of it."

Faith Linked to Better Physical Health

Many patients have a similar reaction when receiving a cancer diagnosis, "Why me?" or they feel like they're being punished. A cancer diagnosis does not have to mean feeling physically terrible though. When people find feelings of transcendence, meaningfulness, or peace they report feeling the least physical problems. The journal Cancer recently published a review of studies involving more than 32,000 cancer patients, where the study found a link between patients with higher levels of religious or spiritual beliefs reporting better physical health. People who have strong faith tend to think in ways that are healthy. Faith gives people a sense of meaning and purpose in life, which is linked to better health.

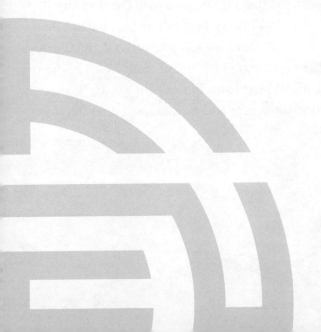

You Are in My Prayers

Spiritual and religious traditions have advocated regular prayer as an essential practice for individual enlightenment and divine connection. This can even include wishing someone else well, as in, "You are in my prayers." Recently, studies have shown that prayer not only prevented people from getting sick but helped them get better faster when they did get sick. Researchers at San Francisco General Hospital looked at the effect of prayer on 393 cardiac patients. Half were prayed for by strangers who only had the patients' names. The patients prayed for had fewer complications, fewer cases of pneumonia, and needed less drug treatment. Studies have also revealed believers recover from breast cancer quicker than non-believers and have better outcomes. Whether used for yourself or for others, prayer is a powerful healing tool available to all.

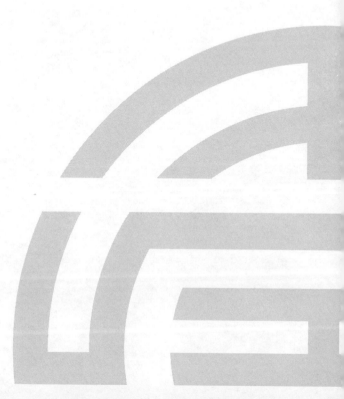

Meditation Leads to Positive Physiological Changes

Meditation is an integral practice in Eastern spiritual and religious traditions. Taoist hermits and Buddhist monks consider meditation as a gateway to enlightenment and healing. And research over the last 10 years has confirmed the belief that meditation practices have physical benefits. A review of cancer patients who used meditation practice showed it to have positive effects on cytokine, an inflammatory protein, thereby helping in the recovery of the immune system. In other words, regular practice of meditation has a restorative action on the immune system.

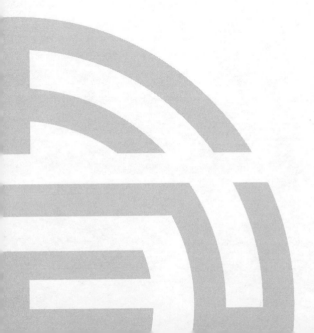

Visualization and Guided Imagery Increased Natural Killer Cells

Visualization practice, or guided imagery, is a technique in which a person imagines and visualizes pictures, sounds, smells, and other sensations associated with accomplishing a goal, such as recovering from illness. At Oregon Health and Science University, a study was conducted on women with stage I and II breast cancer who used guided imagery. Each patient was led through individual guided imagery sessions where the women were encouraged to imagine protective immune cells finding, destroying, and removing cancer cells. After just 8 weeks of practice, researchers found that the women had much less depression and higher natural killer cell counts.

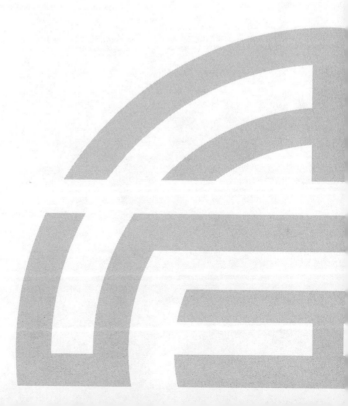

Meditation Improves Treatment Outcome

The overwhelming stress of receiving a cancer diagnosis causes a patient's body to switch to survival mode. This leads to stress hormone and neurochemical imbalance, or hypothalamic–pituitary–adrenal (HPA) axis dysregulation. The HPA axis is your body's stress-coping system. Studies show that HPA dysregulation in cancer patients hastens disease progression and decreases survival time for breast, lung, ovarian, and renal cell carcinoma patients. The good news is that findings suggest that meditation practice during chemotherapy can reduce malfunctions in the stress-coping system. This empowers cancer patients with a self-care technique to improve their treatment outcome.

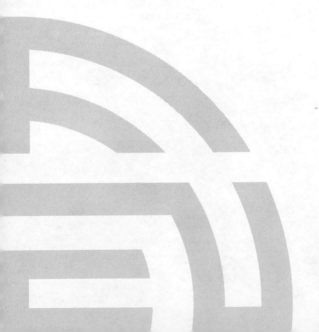

Resilience Improves
Quality of Life in Cancer Survivors

Studies show cancer patients who exhibit resilience had better quality of life during and after cancer treatment. The ability to overcome life and health challenges, move forward from traumatic experiences caused by cancer, and regain meaning and purpose in one's life is called resilience. Resiliency is something that people must actively practice. It is a skill that can be learned and cultivated. It may be innate to some, but that doesn't mean others cannot learn it. Resiliency also means developing a positive outlook, coping skills, and a support system to help neutralize the negative psychological impacts of cancer. Instead of merely surviving, resilient people thrive in their day to day lives.

To develop more resilience, experts agree that you should realize not everything in life can be controlled and focus instead on what you can control and change for the better. Identify stressors, developing strategies to manage or avoid them is essential to effective coping. Reflect on past experiences in order to draw meaning from current situations. Always try to maintain a positive outlook, a cup half full instead of half empty can go a long way toward helping you celebrate little wins. Practice gratitude for what you do have and strive towards healing both your mind and body. And when you can, look for ways to give back and help those who are traveling the same path you once did, by helping others you derive purpose and meaning for your own life.

(The Five Element Personality archetype outlined in the following pages are excerpted from Live Your Ultimate Life by Dr. Mao Shing Ni, published by Tao of Wellness Press)

Five Elements Personality

The Five Elements Personality system has been studied, recorded, and utilized for thousands of years in China. It is used to help doctors advise patients on preventive health and healing, employers hire the right person for a job, and matchmakers pair compatible people in marriage. The secret knowledge of the Five Elements is even more relevant to our complex, ever-changing, modern world today. The wisdom of the Five Elements reveals not just personality dispositions but also physical health and behavioral tendencies that impact all areas of your life, from your health and relationships, to career and finances.

Everyone possesses all five Elements, but there is one core or dominant Element in you that expresses your Element/Personality Type. Each Element possesses unique characteristics of strengths and weaknesses, personality, temperament, and health tendencies. By understanding your core Element and using techniques discussed throughout this book to optimize it, you will be able to remove obstacles and leverage your strength to achieve your full potential.

You Are Authoritative, Confident, and Intense— You Are the Wood Element

As a Wood Element you tend to be highly motivated and have a very strong personality that some identify as Type A. You can appear to be authoritative, confident, intense, smart, decisive, and responsible. A Wood Personality is usually characterized as positive and charismatic. You command respect and make good managers.

If your Wood energy is in balance, you are a charismatic leader, someone who gathers people and makes exciting new things happen. However, you tend to be impatient for people and things to change. When change doesn't happen according to your time-table you become frustrated easily. Remember though that stress comes along with change. If you're unbalanced, the stress will cause your liver network to become stagnant, leading to depression. A careless diet, endless stress, and recreational drugs and alcohol weaken the liver and create a brittle nervous system.

Wood Element corresponds with the liver network in the human body. The intricate arrangement of cells in the liver resembles those in grass and leaves, acting as filters to trap and eliminate toxins in the body. Therefore, Wood Element persons are most vulnerable through their liver. In Chinese medicine, the liver network also encompasses the ability to freely express one's emotions. When feelings are suppressed, or blocked liver network imbalances arise. This leads to physical symptoms like hopelessness, abdominal bloating, indigestion, and resentment.

Don't Let Obstacles Stop You—Go Around It

Your challenge is to learn to readjust after running into an obstacle, rather than becoming angry and frustrated. A healthy Wood personality is like a determined ant; if one direction is blocked, the ant scurries around until it finds another way around the obstacle. A healthy Wood person is flexible yet strong. You listen and learn from others, arrive at a balanced point of view, then push forward with extraordinary creativity and remarkable, forward-moving energy.

To balance your Element, recite or chant the following invocation 36 times daily:

> Divine One of Peace and Tranquility,
> Please help me release my anger,
> Resentment and frustrations.
> I am forever grateful.
> Thank you.

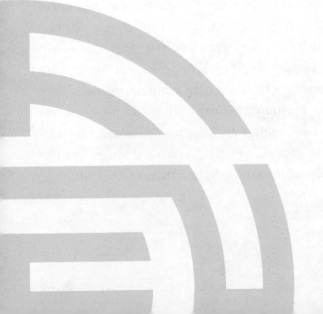

A Joyful, Passionate, and Charismatic Spirit— You Are the Fire Element

A person with strong Fire energy can be very articulate, charismatic, and excel at leadership. Your element commands strong emotional expression and experiences that can yield satisfying results and personal success. It will be helpful to build your leadership skills in order to help others fulfill their goals and dreams. Your special ability to motivate people and inspire their passion is a personal asset that will allow you to joyfully connect with others.

When your Fire energy is out of balance you may be too easily stimulated and excitable and lose attention to details. Your need for feeling fired up can drive you to search for other means of stimulation, potentially causing you to become addicted or dependent on unhealthy habits.

Fire Element is represented in the human body by the heart network. It is said that Fire people literally feel in their hearts. According to Chinese medicine, the heart houses the spirit. And because the heart and spirit are not separable, one of your many attributes is intuition. You can sense other's pain instinctively and feel empathy towards them. Not surprisingly, as a high-energy Fire elemental type, you tend to develop cardiac or circulation problems, high blood pressure, and anxiety.

Passion Has Its Vulnerable Side

As a Fire elemental type, you are able to express feelings passionately that move others, yet you tend to be vulnerable to criticism and your feelings can be easily hurt. You may also possess a strong ego. It is possible that you have a difficult time getting along with others, which ultimately leads to isolation and loneliness. Because of your natural emotional need for acknowledgement and validation, you can easily slip into codependency. You need to learn how to be vulnerable without giving up emotional independence.

To balance your Element, recite or chant the following invocation 36 times daily:

> Dear Divine One of Joy,
> Please help me release the pain and hurt
> and help me let go of my negative attachments.
> I am forever grateful.
> Thank you.

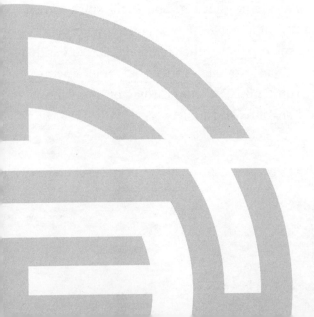

You are Caring, Empathetic, and Nurturing—You Are the Earth Element

Earth Element people tend to be caring, empathetic, and nurturing. Like the earth's bounty that sustains all life, you express your Earth nature through kindness and concern for those around you. Like a mother who nurtures her children with unconditional love, you possess the natural desire to tend to others. You seek first to understand and therefore are empathetic to people's sufferings and misfortunes.

As an Earth person, you are probably thoughtful and generous to a fault. You tend to overcompensate and make up for what is lacking in others. You can easily give more than you receive, and your interpersonal relationships become off balance. Because you are a natural caregiver you may find that you feel drained and exhausted to the point of feeling used, or even resentful.

In Chinese medicine, Earth energy oversees nourishment. Because nourishment for your body depends upon healthy digestion, it is no surprise that a person with unbalanced Earth energy has a tendency toward stomach and digestive issues. Indigestion, bloating, and sugar highs and lows are common in your element, so for you, diabetes could be lurking just around the corner.

Nourish Your Earth Spirit

In Chinese medicine, Earth energy is also responsible for information processing and thought. If you worry, over-think, and obsess while having a poor diet it can throw you completely out of balance. This leads to brain fog, fixation, and rumination. Earth Element oversees nourishment, not only nourishment for your body but also nourishment for your spirit. When your Earth element is in balance, you are a happy, healthy, loving, and giving human being.

To balance your Element, recite or chant the following invocation 36 times daily:

> Dear Divine One of Constancy,
> Please help me release all my worries and anxiety
> and strengthen my foundation.
> I am forever grateful.
> Thank you.

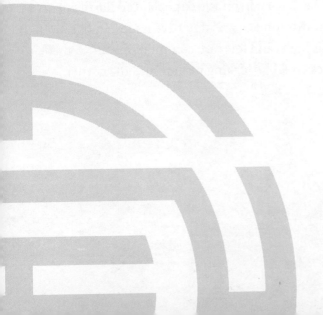

You Are Methodical, Intelligent, and Analytical— You Are the Metal Element

The Metal Element personality tends to be intellectual, inquisitive, and analytical. You naturally excel at taking reams of information that may overwhelm others and organizing them into systematized and accessible arrangements. Transformation is a skill that you readily apply, taking seemingly unrelated parts and assembling them into a unified whole. Additionally, you effortlessly analyze and make sense of complex problems.

If you are an unbalanced, opinionated, inflexible Metal person, it is quite possible that you subscribe to long-held principles and beliefs. As a perfectionist, you can be very critical, both of yourself and of others. Cultivating tolerance and acceptance of your own attributes and those of others is a very important aspect of bringing your element into balance. Whether you perceive these attributes to be positive or negative, your acceptance of them will stop overly critical thinking and help you embrace change and challenge.

Metal Element is represented in the human body by the lung energy network. It is associated with the defense systems of the body, which includes immunity, the intestinal tract, and the skin. The lungs are the body's defense against pathogens. Metal elemental types of people whose energy is weak or unbalanced are prone to respiratory conditions like shortness of breath, stuffiness, sinusitis, allergy, asthma, colds, and flu. Other signs of Metal Element imbalance include cough, dry skin, constipation, colitis, skin breakouts, fatigue, chills, a weak voice, exhaustion, sadness, and self-destructive behaviors.

The Alchemy of Transformation

Transformation is both the nature and symbol of the Metal element. This symbol refers to ancient alchemists who experimented in an effort to transform base metals into gold. The challenge of the Metal personality is self-discovery, followed by cultivation and self-actualization. This transformation can be accomplished through self-cultivation in order to reach the gold of a balanced Metal element. This journey begins by peeling back the protective layers of the personality in order to discover and acknowledge who you are. From there you will discover your potential and finally be able to actualize your goals.

To balance your Element, recite or chant the following invocation 36 times daily:

> Dear Divine One of Great
> Compassion, help me release all my sadness
> and allow me to gain profound
> Understanding of the human condition.
> I am forever grateful.
> Thank you.

You Are Wise, Persistent, and Deep— You Are the Water Element

As a Water element person, you are a confident, powerful force with a great capacity for endurance. Your strong will and confidence is not due to an excessive ego; it comes from a very deep-rooted connection to your very being, your foundation, your Jing or essence. There's depth to the quality of your being, like that of the deep blue sea. It is primal and mysterious.

Water Element is associated with a strong survival instinct motivated by fear. It is quite possible for you to overwork to the point of exhaustion or to become so anxious that you become emotionally paralyzed. Your fear can be balanced with education and knowledge that will help you understand the difference between risk and reward. That way, like Water flowing in nature, you can always find a way around any blockage.

Water regulates the kidney energy network. This includes the bladder, reproductive organs, and the hormonal system. Thus, Water people are susceptible to urinary, hormone, and reproductive problems. The kidney adrenals are particularly vulnerable to stress. Therefore, it is very important for you to cultivate your essence by soaking up the right nutrients, herbs, and supplements.

Transcend the Fear and Keep Flowing

It is natural for your Water energy to have two sides: one side is vulnerable, and the other is fearless. When you are tired, and your energy is out of balance, you may feel a bit cautious and unwilling to take risks even though you are very creative and capable. It is also possible for you to become anxious when you are in situations you cannot control, like flying in an airplane. The solution is for you to learn the facts and then apply your wisdom to any problems that occur.

To balance your Element, recite or chant the following invocation 36 times daily:

> Dear Divine One of Great Courage,
> Please help me release all my fears
> and help me strengthen my will.
> I am forever grateful.
> Thank you.

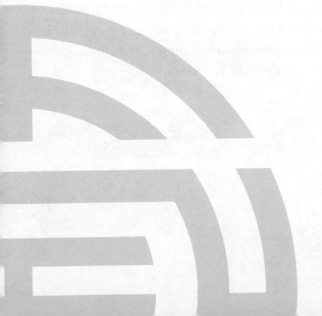

Cultivate a Balanced Personality by Balancing Your Five Elements

Your personality mirrors your core Element. Wood is authoritative, Fire is passionate, Earth is caring, Metal is methodical, and Water is wise. You are born with talents and challenges. Your inherent talent supports and builds your confidence, helping you to meet your challenges. The key to a healthy personality is to understand your core Element, your strengths, your weaknesses, and work on overcoming your challenges so that you are balanced in your Element. Challenges are like rocks that can be either stepping-stones or stumbling blocks. There is no need to be stalled by challenges. The ultimate objective is to cultivate the positive attributes of all Five Elements for a balanced personality. The joy of life is a dance between accepting your gifts and exploring new ones.

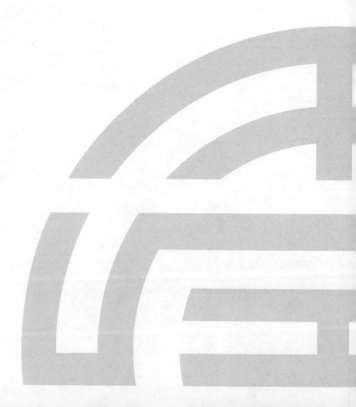

Attaining a Balanced Mind

Most people overly develop their intellectual mind and neglect to nurture their emotional and spiritual mind. Achieving a healthy, well-rounded mind increases your effectiveness in life by building on your intuition and creativity. Positive mental health is about transcending emotions and resolving any entanglements. Your mind is in charge of managing all your affairs and actions. Negative emotions arise when your expectations and belief systems conflict with reality, and you find yourself unable to reconcile the gap. Nurturing the mind will help you respond to any situation appropriately, and help you be free to move beyond your old emotional and behavioral patterns.

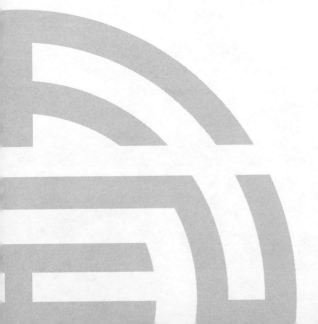

A Healthy Mind Is Key to a Healthy Body

Your mental health is the key to your physical health. As the mind orchestrates all aspects of your worldly life, your physical health greatly impacts your mind. Spiritual health is also largely dependent on the improvement of your mental health, as a peaceful mind enlivens a joyful spirit.

Long ago, Chinese medicine developed practices like qi gong, tai chi, and meditation as ways for people to cultivate a calm and peaceful mind. People often notice that when they practice tai chi or qi gong, they become calmer and more effective in their current tasks. Meditation is another effective way to improve your mind's health as it helps you let go of stale and stuck emotions and allows your mind to become calm and aware. These and other practices nurture intuition and develop spiritual awareness, which gently guides our actions and brings greater peace to our lives.

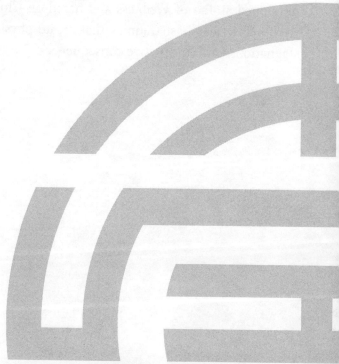

Free Yourself from Emotional Entanglement

Emotions are a natural part of life that communicate and express your inner world. Understanding your emotions can help you to improve and grow, but unhealthy emotions can block you from seeing the truth. You may be a genius when it comes to helping others solve their emotional problems and yet paralyzed by your own. This is because you can be a detached and objective observer when you analyze other people's issues, but often lose that objectivity when you are in the midst of experiencing your own emotional upheaval and turmoil.

A healthy emotional state results in the healing of past traumas, and full acceptance of yourself and others. It provides the vehicle for self-discovery, a deeper connection with others, and a richer life experience. We encourage our patients to explore Acu-Release Technique (ART), a simple but effective trauma release method developed at Tao of Wellness and based on Chinese medicine. ART helps clear past traumas that create physical and energy stagnations with destructive consequences.

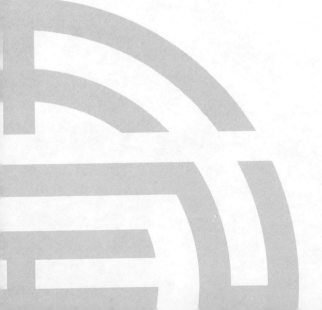

Develop Your Intuition and Creativity

Intuition and creativity are your higher mind; they come from nurturing your subconscious and trusting its expressions. Intellectual learning helps you acquire knowledge, and yet a busy mind filled with excessive knowledge can inhibit the development of intuition and block your access to unlimited resources and creativity. Worse, incessant mental distractions, ceaseless chatter and rumination, and negative emotions all act like a cloud covering the night sky, separating you from your true North. It's easy to see why many people lose their way, never reaching their potential and actualizing their life purpose.

The most effective way to clear these stifling patterns is to nurture self-awareness and a reflective mind. Use contemplation, invocation, and meditation to awaken the power that is inherent within you to help guide and manifest your true life. When you clear the decks and allow yourself adequate time and a peaceful environment, then your native intuition naturally will manifest. If you are interested in cultivating your spirit and your intuition, meditation practices are a helpful way to begin.

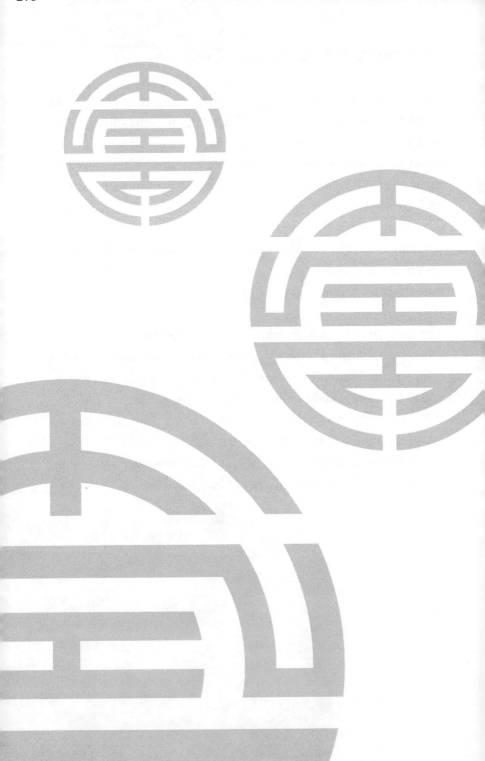

Chapter 8: Where You Are — Environmental Toxins

I am Mother Nature. All of creation bows before me. When people leave their cities and learn of me—walk in my woods, bathe in my rivers, eat of my harvest—they will find healing to their souls. But stray from me and return to the supposed wisdom of men, and they will find themselves in chains once more.

— *Seth Adam Smith*

Since the 1950's, researchers have been studying cancer-causing chemicals and their immunosuppressive properties. These chemicals have come to be known as carcinogens. There have been volumes upon volumes of studies and data collected on carcinogens. Most all of them have a common conclusion: many of the industrial chemicals that have spilled into our environment are endangering both wildlife and human health.

Some examples of items carcinogenic ingredients are found in are:

- Cosmetics
- Toiletries
- Common household products
- Pesticides
- Prescription drugs

And toxins such as dioxins, polychlorinated biphenyls (PCBs), pesticides, and plastics are rampant in our environment. These chemicals, among literally hundreds of thousands of others, are known carcinogens. They weaken one's immune system and subject those exposed to an even greater chance of cancer and other degenerative diseases. Many of these chemicals also cause estrogenic effects in the human body, and in the case of women's bodies, can vastly increase the risk of breast cancer.

When it comes to toxin exposure and accumulation in your body, it's not whether you have been in contact with them or not, but rather at what point do they begin to cause serious damage to your DNA and threaten your health. The troubling fact is that in conventional medicine, there are no available treatments to eliminate toxins such as bisphenol A and flame retardants, two of the most prevalent chemical compounds that exist in everyday life. These toxins can be found in plastic containers, utensils, pajamas, bedding, and more.

This chapter will discuss known carcinogens found in common products. As well, we will advise alternative, healthy substitutes whenever possible and available.

That Water Is Not as Clean as You Thought

There is no doubt water is essential for life. However, the quality of water one consumes matters immensely for one's health. The Environmental Protection Agency estimates that up to 7,000 pollutants exist in both municipal and well drinking water. About 50% of water pollutant exposure is through the skin, with the remainder being through breathing and drinking. Of the many carcinogenic pollutants in water, the most common is trihalomethanes (THMs). THM's can cause liver and kidney damage, as well as nervous system depression and cancer.

Pharmaceutical drugs have been showing up increasingly in municipal water, examples include:
- Anti-seizure
- Anti-depressant
- Oral contraceptives

In addition, heavy metals have been found in water supplies due to metal pipes, asbestos cement, farming runoff, and industrial dumping. A selection of just some are:
- Lead
- Mercury
- Manganese
- Cadmium
- Nickel
- Copper
- Chromium
- Lead
- Zinc
- Aluminum

- Cobalt
- Arsenic

To top it off, the chlorine used to kill microbes in municipal water supplies has spawned chlorine-resistant Giardia and Pseudomonas infections.

Solution: Avoid buying water in plastic bottles which have traveled long distances and may leach PCBs. Use either an over or under the counter, multistage, carbon water filter at home and carry your own drinking water. Use filtered water for cooking and bathing; for showering get a shower head filter. If feasible, install a whole-house filtration system. (See the Resources section for recommendations)

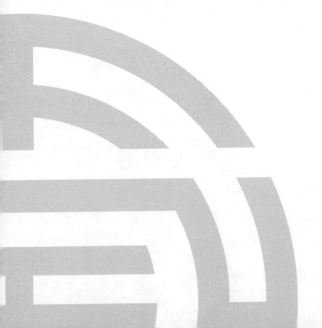

Eat Organic and Avoid Pesticides

US farmers alone use 1.5 billion tons of pesticides and herbicides each year. Examples include oranges wrapped in fungicides, mushrooms fumigated with formaldehyde, and potato and onions treated with maleic hydrazide. Many of these pesticides have been shown to cause cancer, birth defects, and genetic changes in animals. While some of the most toxic ones have been banned in the US, they are still exported to developing countries and make their way back via imported produce.

Solution: Look for foods marked USDA, Food Alliance, Quality Assurance International, and other certified organic produce. These are often found at your local farmers' market, food co-ops, and health food stores. Better yet, if you've got the space and time, grow your own fruits and vegetables for the ultimate peace of mind, as well as emotional and physical satisfaction. If you can't get 100% organic, scrub and rinse produce thoroughly, peel the skin, or try to avoid the top 12 most pesticide-contaminated produce.

The Dirty Dozen, the most pesticide-sprayed foods are:
- Spinach
- Potatoes
- Bell peppers
- Celery
- Lettuce
- Apples
- Strawberries
- Peaches
- Pears

- Nectarines
- Cherries
- Grapes

The Clean Dozen, the least pesticide-sprayed foods include:

- Asparagus
- Cabbage
- Onions
- Eggplant
- Broccoli
- Frozen sweet corn
- Frozen sweet peas
- Avocado
- Pineapple
- Mango
- Kiwi
- Banana

Sulfites Can Compromise Immunity

Sulfites are used to prevent spoilage and discolorations in food in order to extend shelf life. As a result, they are prevalent in both food production and restaurant salad bars, fruits, and seafood. They are commonly used to preserve freshness in:

- Dried fruits
- Soups
- Vegetables
- Salad dressings
- Sauces
- Gravy
- Corn syrup
- Shellfish
- Avocado dips
- Potatoes
- Packaged lemon juice

Look for words like sulfur dioxide, sodium sulfite, and sodium and potassium bisulfite/metabisulfite on packaged food. Except for organic wine, they are almost always used when making beer and wine to control naturally occurring yeast organisms. People with sulfite allergies may develop wheezing, vomiting, diarrhea, hives, and even anaphylactic shock from exposure.

Solution: Whenever possible, avoid packaged foods and fast food. Instead, opt for farmers' markets, health food stores, and restaurants promoting local, sustainable, and organic products.

Stop Nitrates from Becoming Nitrosamine

Sodium nitrite and potassium nitrite are used in 65% of all cheese, pork, poultry, fish, and other meat. They are also prevalent in processed meats such as bacon, sausages, hot dogs, and luncheon meats. They're commonly used to preserve pink color and inhibit bacterial growth in processed meats and cheeses.

When nitrates are combined with amines during meat processing, curing, and cooking they will form nitrosamine. Nitrosamine is highly carcinogenic and may lead to pancreatic, gastrointestinal, and lung cancers. Fried bacon, for example, contains high amounts of nitrosamine. It is also found in cigarettes and drinking water.

Solution: You can greatly reduce or eliminate your exposure to nitrosamine by entirely avoiding:
- Preserved meat
- Salted fish
- Barbeque and burnt meat
- Pickles
- Cigarette smoke

Increasing your intake of natural antioxidants such as garlic, green tea, and vitamin-C-rich fruits and vegetables will effectively suppress nitrosamine formation. For instance, vitamin C can prohibit the formation of nitrosamines in the stomach.

Eating Dyed Salmon or Oranges Is Not What Nature Intended

Ever notice that all the oranges in the supermarket bin are exactly the same color? Even though oranges from the same tree in your yard vary in color? When you see FD&C Yellow #6, Red #3, and Blue #1 and #2 on a food label you'll know instantly that it contains artificial colors. They are used widely and found in:

- Candies
- Pastries
- Cakes
- Beverages
- Packaged snacks
- Fruits
- Farm raised salmon

For instance, green oranges from Florida that are in markets before January are treated with ethylene gas to remove the "green color" from the rind. Afterwards, they are dipped in Red No. 32 to dye them orange.

Another example involves farm raised salmon. Wild salmon's flesh is naturally pink due to eating natural food. On the other hand, the flesh color of farm raised salmon is naturally gray. Therefore, farm raised salmon are dyed pink by "pigmenting" their diet with synthetic or natural colors before being sold. This is in order to make them look more like their wild counterparts.

Solution: Many artificial colors were found carcinogenic in animal studies. Moreover, artificial colors and flavors have been found to cause hyperactivity in children. Therefore, it is best to avoid all artificial food colors. Instead, opt for unadulterated fresh food and, when necessary, use beet, pomegranate, and other juices for natural coloring. An orange is called an orange because of its natural color, not because it's dyed from green to orange.

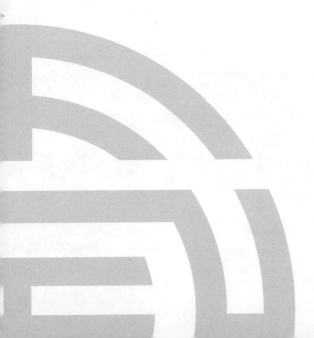

Buy Fresh and in Small Amounts to Avoid the Need for Preservatives

Commercial and industrialized food production in the United States has contributed to the common use of preservatives in foods. They are often used to stop fats from going rancid and preserve freshness. Common additives are:

- Propyl gallate
- Ethylene-diamine tetraacetic acid (EDTA)
- Butylated hydroxyanisole (BHA)
- Butylated hydroxytoluene (BHT)

These are added to:

- Cereals
- Chewing gum
- Vegetable oil
- Potato chips
- Food packaging (to preserve freshness)

They have been found to be carcinogenic in animals and may cause dizziness, sneezing, headaches, nausea, and asthma attacks in individuals.

Solution: I remember growing up in Asia and accompanying my mother to the open produce market almost daily. There we would buy vegetables, fruits, and just-caught fish. By doing this we avoided food preservatives by buying only small quantities of fresh food that we consumed within a few days. For your health's sake, I suggest that you frequent your local farmers market, the same way that our ancestors did.

Growth Stimulants, Hormones, and Antibiotics Are Used Mostly for Animals

In 2013, more than 131,000 tons of antibiotics were used on food animals worldwide. By 2030, it will be more than 200,000 tons. On top of these staggering numbers, consider that in the US alone more than 50% of antibiotics produced go towards animal feed. Virtually 100% of poultry, 90% of pigs and veal calves, and 60% of cattle are fed antibiotics and sulfa drugs. Over 1,000 drugs and another 1,000 chemicals have been approved by the FDA for animal feed, many of which are potential carcinogens, mutagens, and teratogens.

Additionally, many animals are fed artificial colors, hormones, and growth stimulants. Simply by consuming meat and dairy products from bovine somatotropin (bST) treated cows, people are experiencing elevated insulin-like growth factor 1 (IGF-1) and increasing their risk of developing cancer. Another industry practice is adding the arsenic compound roxarsone to chicken feed in order to speed maturation and egg production. This may result in the accumulation of arsenic, a known increaser of cancer risks in humans.

Solution: Try eating a mostly organic, plant-based diet to avoid exposure to growth stimulants and antibiotics used in animal farming. However, if you must eat animal products, insist on grass-fed, organic, free range meats, poultry, and eggs.

Artificial Sweeteners Are Not So Sweet After All

Artificial sweeteners are used to add sweet flavor without the added calories and glucose. At least that's been the reasoning behind beverage makers using them. It turns out, no studies show that artificial sweeteners make any difference in weight management. In fact, more and more studies are showing that daily consumption of sweeteners is associated with a 36% greater risk for metabolic syndrome and a 67% increased risk for type 2 diabetes. Additionally, studies by Italian researchers suggested that high doses of aspartame, one of the most common sweeteners, increased the risk of leukemia and lymphoma in rats.

Despite mounting evidence, the FDA has approved five artificial sweeteners:

- Saccharin
- Acesulfame
- Aspartame
- Neotame
- Sucralose

Moreover, aspartame causes the amino acid phenylalanine to accumulate, especially in people with the disorder phenylketonuria (PKU). This can potentially lead to:

- Seizures
- Brain damage
- Headache
- Mood swings
- High blood pressure
- Insomnia
- ADD and behavioral problems (in children)

Solution: Eat fruit or use its juice as a sweetener in foods. Natural sweeteners with zero or low impact on blood glucose include:

- Stevia
- Monk fruit extract (Luo Han)
- Coconut sugar
- Blackstrap molasses

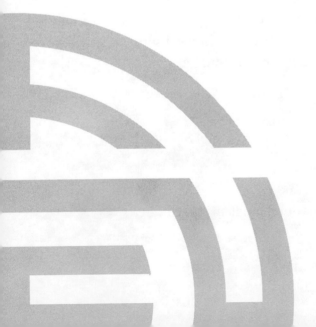

Coal-Tar Containing Dyes Are Toxic for You and Your Unborn Child

Despite having a number of probable carcinogens, hair dyes are exempt from FDA regulation due to a 1938 law. Many contain coal-tar dyes or PPD (para-phenylenediamine), a petroleum-derivative. Research has shown they can lead to cancer when combined with hydrogen peroxide, a common ingredient in hair coloring products. Additionally, ammonia, lead, paragons, and other toxic chemicals are commonly found. Studies conducted on hairdressers found an increase in incidents of bladder cancer, non-Hodgkin lymphoma, leukemia, and breast cancer. And a Consumer Reports investigation found 20 chemicals regularly used in hair coloring that are potential human carcinogens.

Solution: Look for vegetable based hair coloring products, although they don't last as long they contain less toxins. How about trying some homemade non-toxic hair coloring. You can use black coffee or dried sage tea for darker color, lemon juice or turmeric for lighter color. If you are pregnant, wait until you are past the first trimester or 12 weeks before using any hair dyes, and if you do, use the vegetable based ones.

Beware of the Poison Lurking in Your Household Pesticides

Ant, flea, and roach killers, as well as other household pesticides are used in 91% of all US households. They don't just kill unwanted household pests though; they also poison and harm children. The US Poison Control Center reported that over 50% of deaths attributed to pesticides are children. Some household pesticides contain strychnine, parathion, lead arsenate, and other extremely toxic chemicals. These chemicals can store in fatty tissue and accumulate to dangerous levels over time. The warning guidelines for these pesticides speak for themselves:

- "DANGER—poison could kill an adult with a tiny pinch."
- "WARNING—poison could kill with a teaspoon ingested."
- "CAUTION—could kill from 1 ounce to 1 pint ingested."

Solution: Pest-proof your house by keeping it clean, clearing clutter, and storing food properly. Repair leaks, seal cracks, and plant basil and lemon balm around the house to naturally repel insects. Use natural solutions to battle household pests, for instance:

- Repel ants with peppermint and chill.
- Bake your house by turning the heater to maximum and leaving for a day or a weekend to get rid of roaches, silver fish, and fleas.
- Use sticky paper to trap flies and boric acid to kill roaches.
- Put dried bay leaves in grain bins to repel food pests.
- Use vinegar, citronella, or pennyroyal oil to repel mosquitos.
- Mix plaster, flour, and sugar as food to send off the mouse.
- Use natural flea repellent to get rid of fleas.

The Hidden Carcinogens in Clothing, Bedding, and Laundry Cleaners

Most clothes are made in developing countries without the same stringent environmental protection laws as the US. As a result, consumers are being exposed to harmful chemicals and carcinogens from their clothes and bedding. For instance, many fabric dyes contain benzidine, which is cancer-causing. When you sweat these chemicals can be absorbed into the body through your skin. Synthetic fibers contain nylon, polyester, and acrylic which are plastics made from petrochemicals that mimic estrogen and can contribute to elevated risks of breast cancer. Sleep wear, bed sheets, pillows, and mattresses contain flame retardants that studies have shown double the risk of thyroid cancer, especially in women. Additionally, wrinkle-free fabrics contain formaldehyde resins that can irritate skin, sinuses, and eyes. Laundry detergent and bleach often contain compounds that mimic estrogen and can put women at an increased risk of breast cancer. On a positive note, the common dry cleaning agent perchloroethylene (PERC), a confirmed carcinogen, has finally been phased out by the EPA.

Solution: Avoid inexpensive imports that bleed color. Buy clothing, bedding, and mattresses with natural and organic fibers such as cotton, hemp, silk, and wool. Another benefit of silk and wool is that they are naturally flame-resistant, so they contain no flame retardant chemicals. You can use baking soda and borax as natural alternatives to laundry detergent and bleaching agent, respectively. And ask for natural, organic dry cleaning at your local cleaners.

Look out for Radon, Outgas, and Radiofrequency

One of the most common naturally released gases is radon, which is radioactive and the second leading cause of lung cancer. It is found in homes constructed over soil containing radioactive material. Other toxic gases include carbon monoxide, nitrogen dioxide, and hydrogen cyanide from vehicle exhaust. Long term exposure to outgassing from carpets, paints, foam insulation, furniture, and cabinetry made from press-wood boards can cause certain cancers. Additionally, cell phone radiation is considered a possible carcinogen by the World Health Organization.

Solution: Search government databases to find out if your home is within a radon hazard map. Get a HEPA air filter for your bedroom and areas of your home where you spend most of your time. When purchasing furniture or remodeling, avoid particle board with veneer and buy only natural wood furniture and cabinetry. Insist on low or zero VOC, water-based paints. Avoid UFFI (urea-formaldehyde) insulation, seal inside press-wood cabinets, and high VOC areas with foil-backed paper. Keep cell phones at least 6 feet away from your head and use wired earphones instead of wireless sets.

Don't Be a Victim of Sick-Building Syndrome

Modern office and residential buildings are incubators for toxic chemicals and microbes.

These enclosed buildings use HVAC (heating, ventilation, and air conditioning) systems, which re-circulate 75% of the air. In other words, only 25% of the air in the building is fresh. This allows bacteria to stay and breed in the building. If you ever worked in one of these buildings and wondered why everyone got sick so often, this is why. In addition to bacteria, re-circulated air contains contaminants like:

- Volatile organic compounds
- Fiberglass fibers
- Mold
- Fecal bacteria from birds nesting near HVAC equipment
- Bacteria that causes Legionnaires' disease

In fact, studies conducted by OSHA (Occupational Safety and Health Agency) found over 50% of buildings inspected had inadequate air circulation.

Solution: Install HEPA air filtration systems or buy stand-alone units to filter out pollutants from your home and work spaces. Position plants such as indoor ficus, lilies, and palms to absorb toxic gases and return oxygen to the air. And make sure you use full spectrum light bulbs to activate the plants photosynthesis. If possible change your HVAC system's oxygen/fresh air intake settings to more than 50%, clean rooftop HVAC units to prevent debris and moisture from settling in, and change filters frequently.

Cleaning Should be Free of Toxic Chemicals

Common household cleaners contain toxic chemicals.

- Mold and mildew cleaner contain phenol, kerosene, pentachlorophenol, and formaldehyde which are not only cancer-causing but fatal when swallowed.
- Ammonia in glass and all-purpose cleaner can cause injury to lungs, eyes, and skin.
- Rug, carpet, and upholstery shampoo contain perchloroethylene, ethanol, and naphthalene which are carcinogenic and toxic when inhaled.
- Furniture/floor polish contain phenol and nitrobenzene that can cause cancer, genetic changes, birth defects, and organ damage.

Solution: Buy toxin-free cleaning products or make your own.

- Replace ammonia and all-purpose cleaners with vinegar and borax solutions.
- Olive oil and lemon juice make good furniture polish.
- Wipe out mildew, mold, and germs with borax and vodka, and then blow dry with a hair dryer.
- Vinegar and vodka also make very effective glass and window cleaner.
- Clean and deodorize carpet with baking soda.
- Carbonated water, hydrogen peroxide, or vinegar work very well as spot removers.
- Baking soda or table salt are excellent scouring powder for scrubbing your pots and pans.
- Use dried spices, herbs, and essential oils as natural air fresheners.
- Try plain liquid soap and lemon juice to leave your dishes spotless.

Chapter 9: How You Heal — Acupuncture, Herbal Therapy, Bodywork, and Detoxification

Just as the flowers grow from the earth, so the remedy grows in the hands of the physician. The remedy is nothing but a seed that must develop into that which it is destined to be.

—*Paracelsus*

The Hippocratic Oath is taken by every doctor who graduates from medical school. The most common and modern version states, "I will remember that I do not treat a fever chart, a cancerous growth, but a sick human being, whose illness may affect the person's family and economic stability...I will prevent disease whenever I can, for prevention is preferable to cure."

The Hippocratic Oath's focus on both the person who is sick as well as prevention are very much the patient-centered care model of Chinese medicine and prevention. The success of Chinese medicine rests on a naturalistic philosophy of health and healing. It focuses on treating the person, rather than just the disease. Chinese medicine does this by natural means such as diet and nutrition, herbal medicine, acupuncture, bodywork, mind-body exercise, and meditation. Chinese medicine's non-invasive approach and relative lack of side effects, combined with its mind-body approach, has made it an increasingly popular choice as complementary to Western medicine.

Acupuncture has proven to be effective at alleviating cancer symptoms and cancer treatment side effects. It is an evidence-based treatment method used by billions of people worldwide. Besides being an essential adjuvant to cancer treatments, acupuncture has also been found to help in other ways. It helps restore and balance production of serotonin, dopamine, and endorphins. This helps lower levels of anxiety and depression while elevating mood, especially for cancer patients and survivors seeking to prevent recurrence.

Below is the concluding statement from an Acupuncture for Cancer Symposium held recently by the National Cancer Institute (NCI).

"Acupuncture when used with conventional treatment for cancer-related pain have shown better outcomes in pain reduction. Pain reduction in aromatase inhibitor-associated arthralgia is also very positive. Other cancer related symptoms such as fatigue, nausea and vomiting have also shown to be effective in mitigating symptoms. The prevention and treatment of xerostomia are also being studied. As more research is being conducted, the evidence is expanding, leading to the use of acupuncture as a vital part of cancer management protocols.

The need to educate all participants from primary care providers, oncologists, patients and acupuncturists to integrate Western and Eastern is critical in achieving the best outcomes when diagnosed with cancer and health care insurance coverage needs to be made available to make acupuncture available for oncology patients across socioeconomic strata."

We couldn't agree more with the NCI's conclusion!

For many of our patients, their weekly or twice-weekly acupuncture sessions are what they look forward to. It's what sustains and keeps them on track with their chemotherapy and radiation treatments. The best part of acupuncture is that it's free of side effects and directly contributes to increased quality of life. That's what cancer patients need. The feeling that "normal" can be experienced, even while living and coping with a disease that feels so frightening, is of the utmost importance. It gives patients a lifeline and hope to fight on, to not just survive but to thrive.

Herbal medicine has a long history in China, Asia, and the West. In the West, during the Greek era of Hippocrates, herbal therapy was the main method of treatment, much like the role herbal medicine plays in China today. Many modern drugs were originally derived from botanical sources. Some examples are digoxin from the foxglove plant, aspirin from white willow bark, and even the chemo agent Taxol came from the Pacific Yew tree. The main difference between natural herbs and synthesized drugs is how they work. Herbs typically have a slower but holistic effect, while drugs have a faster and targeted action on a specific part or process of the body. Drugs, therefore, have an immediate impact on the symptoms of a disease. However, that immediate gratification comes with a price in the form of unpleasant and sometimes intolerable side effects.

One advantage of the slower, holistic herbal approach is they are mostly free of side-effects. This is ideal for long term prevention use, especially the superior grade herbs in Chinese medicine. Superior grade herbs are sometimes called "tonic" herbs and used mainly to nourish one's body and increase vitality. Many herbs in this category have immune-modulating, antioxidant, and anti-aging properties. Some of the superior grade herbs, such as astragalus root, schisandra berry, and Siberian ginseng are adaptogens. Adaptogens possess properties that help the immune system learn and adapt quickly to changes and environmental stressors so that the body doesn't get thrown off balance.

Adaptogenic herbs are critical in cancer prevention. This is because it is only when the immune system is off balance that renegade cells are allowed to proliferate unchecked. These herbs contain high levels of vitamins and nutrients that are not commonly found in regular foods. Superior grade herbs can be taken for long periods of time, just like food, and without any negative effect. This is why they are also called "food" herbs. They are also used for general prevention of diseases. This chapter will discuss commonly available superior herbs, as well as how to create a customized program incorporating these herbs into one's cancer prevention program. We will also discuss herbs that help patients cope with the side effects of chemotherapy and radiation, as well as aid in recovery from surgery. Ideally, to achieve the full potential of Chinese herbal therapy, we advise that you consult an experienced and licensed practitioner of Chinese medicine.

Bodywork and massage are not only feel-good treatments, they also exert benefits both for general health and dealing with cancer recovery. Chinese medical massage, called tuina, is a specialized medical bodywork for acute muscle and joint injuries, as well as chronic inflammation and pain. It has the wonderful ability to help you relax when you are under stress and feeling tense or anxious. Tuina bodywork is also prescribed for mental and physical detoxification. Tuina bodywork enhances acupuncture because it prepares the body and mind by opening the bioelectric communication pathways. When combined, both acupuncture and bodywork can reduce the healing time for most any condition.

Chinese medicine has long recognized the need to lower cancerous toxins in the body through sweating, urination, and defecation. At the Tao of Wellness, we have designed a unique bodywork protocol to successfully eliminate heavy metals, BPA, flame retardants, and other carcinogenic chemicals. The Tao of Wellness Detox Protocol consists of five steps:

1. Dry skin brushing to exfoliate dead skin cells and stimulate the release of toxins through the skin.
2. Manual therapy along lymphatic vessels to help clear out toxins for elimination.
3. Whole-body cupping to bring blood and body fluids to the surface for easy release of toxins.
4. Infrared heat therapy, which employs infrared light to induce sweating and expel toxins. This is combined with vegetable juicing, hydration, and electrolyte supplementation.
5. Acupuncture treatment to stimulate and support the detoxification actions of the liver, kidney, lungs, and skin, as well as boosting immunity.

The results have been highly satisfying for patients.

Speaking of heat therapy. Research has shown that high temperatures can damage and kill cancer cells, usually with little to no injury to normal tissues. This is known as hyperthermia, a type of treatment in which body tissue is exposed to high temperatures (up to 113°F). It works by killing cancer cells and damaging proteins and structures within cells. The National Cancer Institute (NCI) recommends the inclusion of hyperthermia with chemotherapy and radiation treatments. Evidence has shown improved outcomes with concurrent use.

After 30 years of clinical experience, we have found the combined use of Western and Chinese medicine to be the most beneficial for cancer treatment. The dual approach allows patients to fully benefit from the cancer-killing properties of chemotherapy and radiation, while keeping side effects to a minimum and maintaining a good quality of life. Chinese herbal therapy has not only been proven safe, in a number of cases it has been shown to be synergistic and complementary to chemotherapy. It's a winning strategy that places patients above everything else.

In this chapter, we will provide evidence of the efficacy of the various therapies employed by Chinese medicine. You will learn how they can be part of your integrative cancer management and prevention strategy.

Acupuncture Reduced Hot Flashes in Woman with Breast Cancer

Acupuncture has been used effectively to treat hot flashes in healthy postmenopausal women. It also helps women post-surgery. A Norwegian study was conducted on women taking tamoxifen after breast cancer surgery. These patients found acupuncture reduced their hot flashes both during the day and at night by almost 60%. No corresponding changes were seen in the control group.

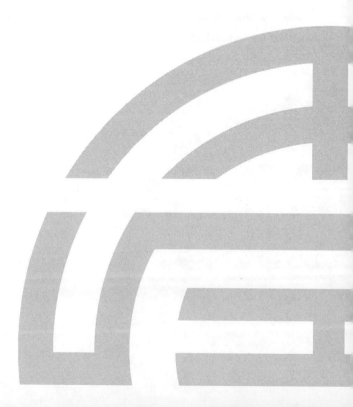

Acupuncture Is a Valuable Adjunctive Treatment for Bone Pain

Bone pain is the most common type of pain caused by cancer. Bone metastases are common in advanced cancers, particularly in:

- Multiple myeloma
- Breast
- Prostate
- Lung

Current pain relieving strategies include the use of opioid-based painkillers, bone density drugs, and radiotherapy. Although patients experience some pain relief, these interventions may produce unacceptable side-effects which inevitably affect the quality of life. Studies show that acupuncture presents a potentially valuable adjunct to existing pain relief strategies. It is also known to be relatively free of harmful side-effects.

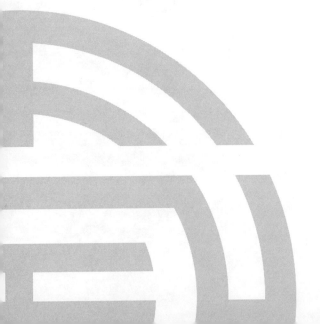

Moxibustion Along with Acupuncture Improved Bone Marrow Function

Leukopenia, or low white blood cells (WBC), is a common side effect of chemotherapy. This is due to the chemo drugs suppression of bone marrow function. White blood cells are produced in the bone marrow and are important to your immune function. Low levels of WBC is indicative of low bone marrow activity. The Yellow Emperor's Classic of Medicine gives one preventive remedy for "maintaining healthy resistance against pathogens." It says to burn the herb mugwort to heat and stimulate a specific acupoint known as stomach 36, located just outside of and below the knee cap. This treatment type is known as moxibustion.

In a study of 386 medium and advanced-stage cancer patients with chemotherapy-induced leukopenia, moxibustion and acupuncture increased the WBC count in 38% of the patients. In another study, 121 patients with leukopenia during radiation and chemotherapy underwent daily acupuncture and moxibustion treatments. After 5 days, their white blood cell counts increased.

Acupuncture May Stimulate Anticancer Immunity

A number of studies have shown acupuncture stimulates an increase in natural killer (NK) cell quantity and function. Researchers from the University Of California Department of Medicine concluded that acupuncture induces a significant increase in NK cell tumor-killing activity, as well as secretion of interleukin-2 (IL-2) and interferon-γ (IFN-γ) in the spleen. Both IL-2 and IFN-γ stimulate the immune system to target cancer cells. Since NK cells are immune cells known to play a key role in killing cancer cells and regulating anticancer immunity, acupuncture may directly contribute to the enhancement of conventional oncology treatments.

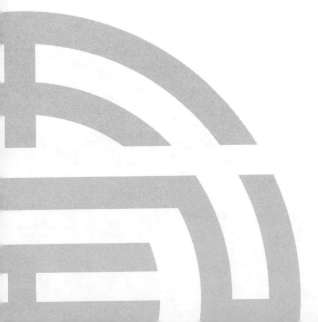

Acupuncture Is a Useful Treatment for Lymphoedema

Lymphoedema is a distressing problem which causes swelling in the body and affects many women after breast cancer surgery. There is no cure and existing treatments are marginally beneficial, rarely reducing swelling in any meaningful way. Researchers from Memorial Sloan-Kettering Cancer Center studied acupuncture as a treatment for women with chronic lymphedema after breast surgery. They found acupuncture reduced the severity of lymphoedema, while causing no serious harmful events during or after treatment. Their conclusion? Acupuncture appears safe and may reduce lymphoedema associated with breast cancer surgery.

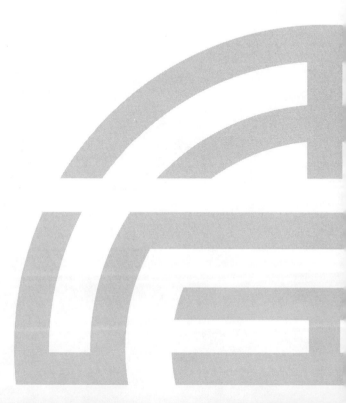

Acupuncture Drastically Reduced the Need for Anti-Nausea Medication

In Germany, a study was conducted on children receiving chemotherapy for solid malignant tumors. The children were randomly assigned to receive acupuncture treatment during either the second or third chemotherapy course, along with standard anti-nausea medication. For the acupuncture group, the need for nausea and vomit medication was significantly lower compared to the control group. The episodes of vomiting were also significantly lower in the acupuncture group. No side effects occurred and the patients' acceptance of acupuncture was high.

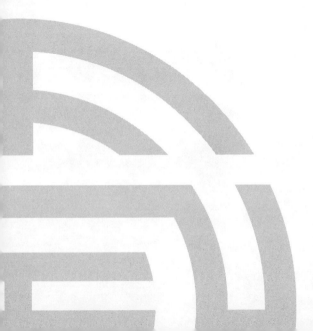

Acupuncture Is Effective for Pain Relief After Cancer Surgery

Researchers at the University of California, San Francisco wanted to know the effects of acupuncture and massage for postoperative symptoms in cancer patients. They conducted a trial assessing the effect of massage and acupuncture combined with usual care, compared to usual care alone. The patients undergoing surgery were randomly assigned to receive either usual care alone or usual care in addition with massage and acupuncture on postoperative days 1 and 2. The patients were followed over the course of three days. The researchers' conclusion: providing massage and acupuncture in addition to usual care resulted in decreased pain and depressive mood among postoperative cancer patients when compared with usual care alone.

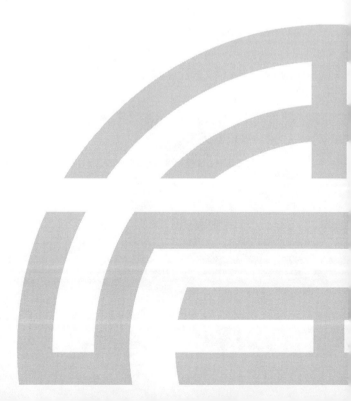

Acupuncture Significantly Reduced Dry Mouth in Radiation Patients

Dry mouth (or xerostomia) after head/neck radiation therapy is a common problem among cancer patients, and conventional medicine is of little benefit. A study published in the journal Cancer featured a trial among patients with nasopharyngeal carcinoma. The study compared acupuncture to standard care in patients who underwent radiation treatment. The result was that acupuncture given concurrently with radiotherapy significantly reduced dry mouth and improved quality of life.

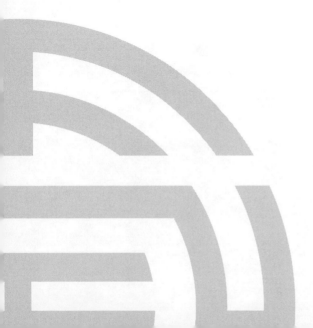

Acupuncture Partially Prevents Chemo-Induced Low White Blood Cell Count

Several clinical trials of patients with non–small cell lung cancer and nasopharynx cancer undergoing chemotherapy have been conducted. They have found that acupuncture could be effective at partially preventing bone marrow suppression-related leukopenia in patients undergoing chemotherapy. This is because the white blood cell (WBC) count in the study group ends up significantly higher than that in the control group

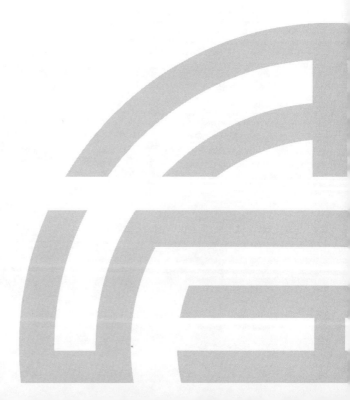

Acupuncture Reduced Insomnia and Improved Melatonin Secretion

A study published in the journal Neuropsychiatry has found acupuncture significantly reduces insomnia and anxiety in study subjects. In addition, the study found that it improved secretion of nocturnal melatonin. This was measured by urine and sleep study measures. Cancer patients are predisposed to insomnia and anxiety due to their illness and side effects of treatments. Therefore, acupuncture is a viable alternative to or adjunct to sleep or anti-anxiety medications.

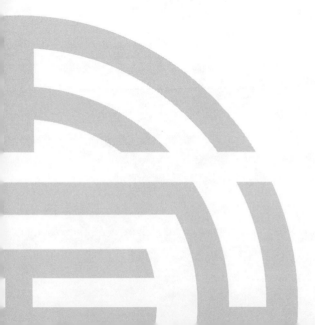

Acupuncture Treatment
Improves Peripheral Neuropathy

Many people suffer numbness, pain, and tingling in their hands and feet following cancer treatment, especially after chemotherapy. The nerve discomfort can interfere with sleep, mood, and equilibrium. This often leads to chronic pain, insomnia, depression, and falls. Patients with neuropathy have been turning to acupuncture to relieve their chronic pain. The results have been promising. Besides relief of pain and numbness, acupuncture also stimulates blood flow to repair nerve damage.

Though ongoing research is being conducted on acupuncture for peripheral neuropathy, there have been some successful studies. One showed that 76% of those who received acupuncture had improved symptoms, versus the only 15% in the control group who received no acupuncture. These findings parallel our clinical experience that there is a positive effect of acupuncture on peripheral neuropathy.

Acupuncture Is Extremely Safe and Well Tolerated

Patient safety is defined as freedom from accidental injury. Acupuncture has been shown as a safe procedure with minimal risk of serious adverse events. In fact, acupuncture would fall into the category of ultra safe practices, according to the patient safety movement in the US. A survey of 12 studies on more than a million treatments reported "the risk of a serious adverse event with acupuncture is estimated to be 0.05 per 10,000 treatments, and 0.55 per 10,000 individual patients." The conclusion was that the risk of serious harm happening due to acupuncture is so low would be below that of many common medical treatments.

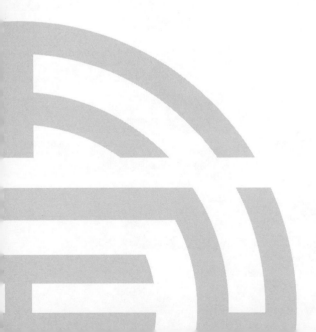

Acupuncture Is Focused on the Patient as a Whole

Patients in the West have increasingly demanded that health care providers respect and tailor treatments to the patient's values, preferences, and needs. The use of acupuncture for cancer patients fulfills these needs. Acupuncture and Chinese medicine is considered a patient-centered practice because it takes into consideration a person's unique constitution, as well as their emotional and physical needs. It provides physical comfort, pain relief, and relaxation during treatment. In addition to its therapeutic benefits, it provides emotional support through patient education and empowerment.

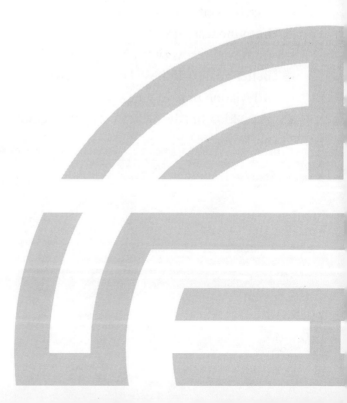

Chinese Herbal Medicine Relieves Chemo Side Effects and Improves Quality of Life

Patients who received Chinese herbal medicine combined with conventional Western treatment during their cancer treatment demonstrated significantly better survival and/or disease response as well as better quality of life than patients receiving Western treatment alone.

This was the conclusion of a literature review performed by the University of Texas Center for Alternative Medicine Research. It compiled many Chinese studies, including controlled trials with human and animal subjects, and test tube laboratory experiments. The studies showed the positive impact of medicinal herbs on:

- Disease response
- Survival outcome
- Immune response
- Improved recovery from surgery
- Better quality of life
- Alleviation of pain
- Reduction in adverse effects from chemotherapy and radiation

Herbal Formulas Are Compounded to Maximize Synergism

Chinese medicine has long recorded not just the therapeutic properties of an individual herb but the enhanced synergistic action of combining herbs into a formula. In other words, the whole formula of many herbs has a greater effect than the sum of its individual herbs. Modern research has confirmed and adopted this. Synergistic principals are now used in pharmaceutical and clinical environments, whether for modern drugs or traditional formulas.

Chinese herbal formulas typically contain 8-15 ingredients and are comprised of four distinct parts.
- Monarchs are principal ingredients that target the immediate cause and symptoms of the disease.
- Ministers enhance the monarch's effects and also target underlying symptoms.
- Assistants treat secondary symptoms, eliminate toxins, and optimize the effects of the other herbs.
- Guides help deliver ingredients to targeted areas.

It takes a trained physician of Chinese medicine at least ten years of clinical practice to master the art and science of herbal formulas. In addition, cures in the form of secret herbal formulas have been passed down from father to son in medical families to ensure the survival and exclusivity of the knowledge.

PHY906 Demonstrated the Power of Synergy in Herbal Formula

A study published in Cancer Chemotherapy and Pharmacology explored the synergic effect of herbal formulas for advanced pancreatic cancer (APC). Currently, APC is treated with the chemo agent gemcitabine. If patients fail to respond to it, there is no standard alternate chemo drug. The study explored the combined use of an ancient Chinese herbal formula named PHY906 with gemcitabine as a second line treatment for APC. PHY906 is comprised of four herbs:

- Scutellaria baicalensis (huang qin)
- Glycyrrhiza (licorice)
- Ziziphus jujuba (jujube date)
- Paeonia lactiflora (white peony)

This herbal formula has been used for over 1,700 years in China and Japan to treat a variety of ailments such as:

- Abdominal cramps
- Fever
- Headache
- Vomiting
- Thirst
- Diarrhea

The analysis showed that the PHY906 formula helped in numerous ways. It boosts the cellular performance of chemotherapy agents by preventing MDR (multi-drug resistance) mechanisms. It adjusts genes responsible for both the innate and adaptive immune response. It inhibits enzymes involved in tumor cell metastasis. Lastly, it discourages angiogenesis or formation of new blood vessels. In other words, PHY906, with its multi-herb components, exerted synergistic action as a whole greater than the sum of its individual herbs. In conclusion, it could be safely used with chemo drugs to enhance a patient's outcome.

Even with the best supportive care, the average survival rate of patients who have failed gemcitabine is approximately two months. That is why this study is so significant. It showed that concurrent use of gemcitabine and PHY906 tripled the average survival time and dramatically reduced side effects such as nausea, diarrhea, and fatigue. The study's author concluded that nearly half of patients with gemcitabine-pretreated disease may be candidates for further treatment with this combination.

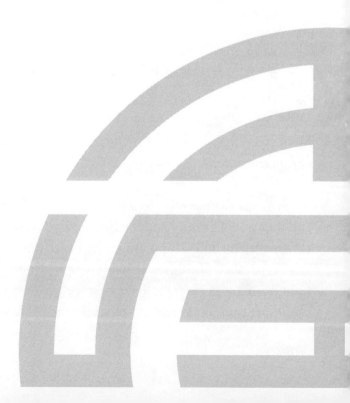

Frankincense Holds Promise for Cancer Prevention

The resin frankincense has been prized in aromatherapy for at least two thousand years by the ancient cultures of China, India, and Egypt. Most people know frankincense from the bible, which says it was delivered to Jesus as an offering from one of the three wise men. Now, researchers from Baylor University Medical Center have found that frankincense helps regulate gene expression, and they believe that it may be effective for both cancer prevention and treatment. Additional studies by University of Leicester researchers indicated that frankincense contains the compound acetyl-11-keto-beta-boswellic acid (AKBA). AKBA targets cancer cells, particularly:

- Ovarian
- Brain
- Breast
- Colon
- Pancreatic
- Prostate
- Stomach

More research is underway to understand the clinical application of frankincense.

Apply Frankincense oil directly onto the skin of the affected area and then add a heating pad for 10-15 minutes. Additional application sites include acupoints in the inner thigh just above the knee cap, called Sp 10 or xue hai. There is also the web between thumb and index finger called LI 4 or he gu. These acupoints are traditionally used to break up blockages and stagnations.

Fu Zheng Therapy: Principles and Practice

Chinese medicine experienced a renaissance in China in the 1950s due to a national mandate by Mao Zedong. This fueled modern clinical research in China and Japan, specifically for searching for ways to improve outcomes for cancer patients undergoing chemotherapy and radiation. This approach came to be known as Fu Zheng Therapy. Over the last three decades, Fu Zheng has become the standard practice of integrative oncology in China.

Fu Zheng means to optimize and restore what is normal. Chinese herbs used in Fu Zheng therapy support non-specific resistance and are known as biological response modifiers, or adaptogens. In 1981, the Academy of Traditional Chinese Medicine in Beijing released a statement on the use of Fu Zheng herbs for cancer patients,

...the treatment of malignant tumors with combined methods of traditional Chinese medicine and western medicine has made much progress...patients with advanced malignant tumors usually are depleted in their blood and life force and suffered declines in the function of their viscera.

Fu Zheng herbs may improve the viscera and the immune function of the patients, enhance resistance against disease, and prolong their survival period. Furthermore, Fu Zheng herbs also have protective effects against immune suppression, lowering of white blood cell count, suppression of bone marrow, and decrease of plasma cortisol levels induced by radiotherapy and chemo-therapy. All this benefits the treatment of malignant tumors.

Fu Zheng Therapy Research in the United States

According to researchers from the University of California, San Francisco,

Fu Zheng therapy produces possible diverse biologic effects that include reduce the tumor load; prevent recurrence or formation of a new primary cancer; bolster the immune system; enhance the regulatory function of the endocrine system; protect the structure and function of internal organs and glands; strengthen the digestive system by improving absorption and metabolism; protect bone marrow and hematopoietic function; and prevent, control, and treat adverse side effects caused by conventional treatments for cancer.

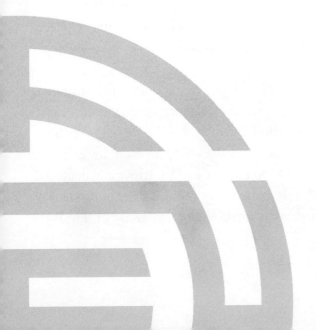

Anticancer Properties of Chinese Herbs

A study published in the journal Anticancer Research analyzed 71 Chinese herbs that have traditionally been used for cancer and confirmed their anti-cancer properties. The anticancer compounds found in Chinese herbs are comprised of various types of phytocompounds (plant compounds) including:

- Alkaloids
- Flavonoids
- Terpenoids
- Anthraquinones
- Polyphenols
- Organic acids
- Polysaccharides
- Saponins

And more.

Other studies indicated that the active compounds from Chinese herbs exhibited multiple anticancer properties, such as:

- Inhibition of proliferation, invasion, and metastasis
- Anti-inflammatory
- Anti-oxidation
- Anti-angiogenesis, which prevents new blood vessel formation

Ultimately, many Chinese herbs have been found to possess actions which positively adjust the immune system, ensuring optimum health function and disease prevention.

Astragalus Increases Vitality and Boosts Immune Function

Astragalus, or huang qi, is the most commonly used Fu Zheng herb for cancer care and prevention. Traditionally, its main action is supporting wei qi, or the immune barrier. This means it increases stamina, strength, and vitality while also boosting immune function against pathogens and abnormal cell growth. Considered an adaptogen, astragalus has antioxidant, anti-inflammatory, and antiviral activities. Anti-cancer properties have also been observed in test tube tests, with some compounds from astragalus working against gastric, colon, liver, and ovarian cancers. Astragalus has also been associated with prolonged survival times in acute myeloid leukemia patients. Studies also showed that when used in combination with the herb ligustri lucidi, astragalus increased survival rates in people who were receiving conventional treatment for breast cancer.

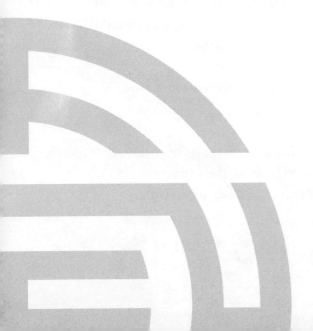

Astragalus Reduces Fatigue, Nausea, and Vomiting in Chemotherapy Patients

Studies also suggest synergistic effects when astragalus is used with chemotherapy. It has been found to enhance chemotherapy and protect against the side effects of the drug oxaliplatin.

Astragalus reverses the toxicity of the drug 5-fluorouracil (5FU). It also enhances the therapeutic benefit of the medication vinblastine, while reducing its red and white blood cell damaging side effects. A study published in Carcinogenesis showed astragalus has anti-tumor, apoptotic (programmed cell death), and inhibited cell proliferation characteristics. These findings show that using astragalus as an adjuvant along with conventional treatment can help reduce cancer-related fatigue and chemo-induced nausea and vomiting.

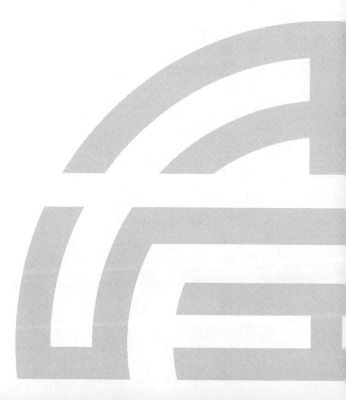

Ligustri Induces Apoptosis in Liver Cancer Cells

The fruit extract Fructus Ligustri Lucidi is a Fu Zheng herb used in traditional Chinese medicine to treat many conditions. Research published in the journal Oncology Reports examined how Ligustri influenced apoptosis, or programmed cell death, in cancer cells located in the liver. The evidence suggests that Ligustri may be a potential adjuvant herb in anticancer therapy.

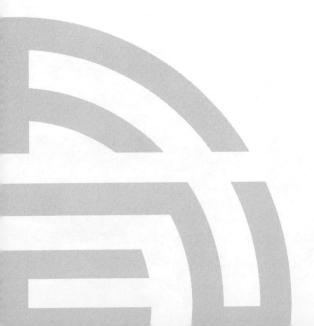

Ginseng Enhances Anti-Tumor Effects in Conjunction with Chemotherapy

A highly regarded Fu Zheng Chinese herb, ginseng has enjoyed an almost mythical status in Chinese culture due to its magic elixir-like properties. A review of ginseng and chemotherapy drug combinations was published in the journal Evidence-Based Complementary and Alternative Medicine. The review concluded that ginseng enhanced anti-tumor effects when used in combination with some chemo drugs.

Ginseng was also confirmed to have excellent potential as a chemotherapy adjuvant because of its low toxicity and many beneficial properties, such as:

- Antiangiogenesis
- Antiproliferation
- Anti-inflammation
- Antioxidation
- Apoptosis
- Immune modulation effects

There are ongoing clinical studies to enhance the applicability of ginseng and other anticancer drugs. This may lead to a wider use of ginseng in cancer treatments.

Atractylodes Supports Metabolic and Digestive Functions

Bai Zhu, or atractylodes, is another Fu Zheng herb that's commonly used during and after cancer treatments. It helps support metabolic and digestive functions while expelling dampness. Dampness in the body happens when excess moisture does not burn off, and it can lead to tumor formation.

A study published in the Journal of Experimental and Clinical Cancer Research demonstrated the anti-tumor effects of atractylodes on bladder cancer cells, both within the human body and in lab experiments. It was found that atractylodes suppressed tumor growth, triggered cell cycle arrest, induced apoptosis, and blocked tumor signaling pathways. The conclusion by the researchers was that atractylodes has the potential to be an acceptable adjuvant therapy to treat bladder cancer alongside conventional treatment.

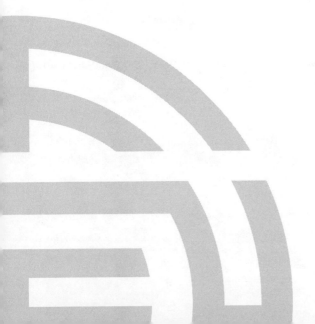

Atractylodes Is Rich in Cancer Fighting Terpenoids

Sesquiterpenes are a class of naturally occurring molecules found in atractylodes. They have shown therapeutic potential in decreasing the progression of cancer and have been considered by researchers as a potential anticancer agent. This is supported by the fact that atractylodes has been part of anticancer herbal formulas in Chinese medicine since around the time of Christ.

In the journal Medical Science Monitor, researchers published a study on the anti-tumor effects of atractylenolide. Atractylenolide is another terpene isolated from atractylodes that has been found to have a positive inhibitory effect on human ovarian cancer cells. The study indicated that atractylenolide can influence cell cycle arrest and apoptosis by preventing tumor signaling pathways in ovarian cancer. These findings warrant the use of atractylenolide as an adjuvant care.

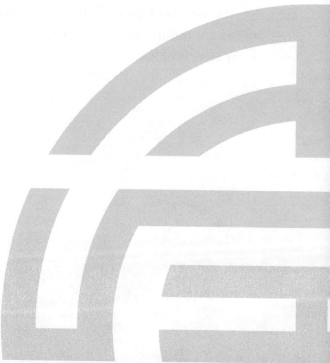

Poria for Stronger Immune Function and Glucose Balance

Poria cocos, or Fu Ling, has been used for thousands of years in Chinese medicine for its diuretic, sedative, and strengthening effects. It is a type of mushroom that is rich in polysaccharides and terpenoids. A study published in Planta Medica showed that Poria may help boost immune function and help fight inflammation. The compounds found in Poria have been shown to help regulate blood sugar levels and treat insulin resistance in subjects, according to another study from Evidence-Based Complementary and Alternative Medicine.

Several studies on human cells showed that Poria suppressed the growth and invasiveness of pancreatic and breast cancer cells. One of the studies was published in the International Journal of Oncology, and the author was able to show the mechanism that targeted "the invasive behavior" of the human pancreatic cell line. Studies are continuing to further the understanding of the anti-cancer aspects of Poria.

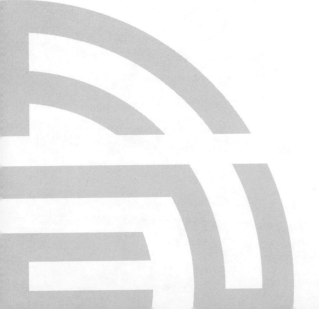

Scutellaria Barbata Slows Proliferation of Breast and Prostate Cancer

The root of Scutellaria barbata, known as Ban Zhi Lian, is an herb long used in traditional Chinese medicine for its anticancer property. A study published in the journal Cancer Biology and Therapy showed how the compounds in Scutellaria inhibited tumor growth in breast and prostate cancer cells. This and other studies show the potential of Scutellaria as an adjuvant herb for integrative cancer care.

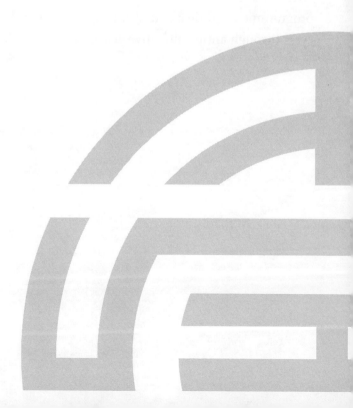

Oldenlandia Inhibits Growth of Cancer Cells

Oldenlandia diffusa is a slender plant found in East Asia and Southern China that resembles a snake. It is also known as Bai Hua She Cao or white snake grass, and has been used in Chinese medicine for cancer treatment for over a thousand years. It is used in traditional Chinese medicine for the treatment of liver diseases, snake bites, and tumors. Laboratory studies suggest that this herb may inhibit the growth of cancer cells and kill them by causing programmed cell death. Studies also show that it may stimulate the immune system to destroy or engulf tumor cells.

A study in the Journal of Ethnopharmacology investigated how Oldenlandia promoted cell death in leukemia cells (HL60) and human lymphocytes. The findings showed that Oldenlandia was effective at inhibiting the growth of leukemia cells and induced programmed cell death. It also affected human blood lymphocytes through antiproliferative actions.

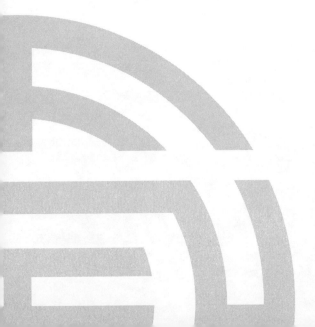

Reishi Mushroom Improves Immune Response and Quality of Life

Reishi, or Ling Zhi, is a medicinal mushroom used in traditional Chinese medicine to promote health and longevity. It is traditionally used to relieve fatigue, reduce inflammation, increase stamina, and support the immune system. In modern times, it is also being used to maintain balance of cholesterol and blood pressure. Reishi contains complex sugars known as beta-glucans, studies suggest that these compounds may help stop the growth and spread of cancer cells.

Investigations into the anticancer effects of reishi have been performed in both lab and human vivo studies. According to a study published in Nutrition and Cancer, immune response and healthy cell division was seen in cancer patients who used reishi. This was reported in one nonrandomized and two randomized trials, and another study observed improved quality of life in lung cancer patients.

Cordyceps Increases Endurance and Performance

Chinese Olympic athletes have enjoyed an edge over others due to supplementing with an herb called cordyceps, or Dong Chong Xia Cao. A study published in the Journal of Alternative and Complementary Medicine showed daily intake of cordyceps improved exercise performance and endurance in a small group of older adults. Its other benefits include improved brain function, lowered insulin resistance, and increased antioxidant activity in aging mice.

Preliminary studies show promise of using cordyceps for certain cancers. One study found that cordyceps may help increase immune defense against breast cancer. Another study presented research on the anti-cancer effects of cordyceps in human colorectal carcinoma RKO cells, showing that the growth of RKO cells was significantly delayed by treatment with cordyceps. Additionally, cordyceps possess exceptional anti-cancer components that are shown to be harmful to colorectal carcinoma RKO cells. Further investigations into using cordyceps as an adjuvant in conventional cancer treatment are ongoing.

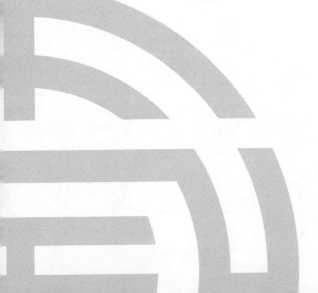

Baicalein Found Useful as an Adjunct Therapy for Liver Cancer

Huang Qin or Scutellaria baicalensis (not to be confused with Scutellaria barbata) is a Chinese herb that is traditionally used for its anti-cancer, anti-bacteria, anti-viral, and anti-allergenic properties. It also contains a flavonoid compound called baicalein that has been found to possess potent anticancer properties. A study published in the journal Biomedicine & Pharmacotherapy provided evidence that baicalein has strong anti-cancer functions against liver cancer cells. Baicalein's mechanisms include:

- Antiproliferation
- Remodel process
- Apoptosis
- Autophagy, or self-devouring cellular recycling

Because of the high mortality rates associated with conventional treatments for advanced liver cancer, researchers conclude that baicalein should be used as an adjunct therapy.

Licorice Protects the Liver Against the Harmful Effects of Chemotherapy Drugs

There are so many powerful herbs found in nature that contain powerful cancer-healing properties. With over 400 compounds in one small root, licorice, also called glycyrrhiza and gan cao, can definitely be considered one of them. Some researchers and doctors recommend that individuals with hormone-sensitive cancers (such as breast, ovarian, uterine, and prostate cancer) avoid using licorice altogether. However, this advice is in direct contrast with recent studies. These new studies have found specific tumor-reducing, immune-boosting, and hormone-regulating compounds within licorice root.

Researchers at the University Sains School of Medical Sciences in Kelantan, Malaysia discovered three different bioactive immunomodulators within licorice. These include:
- Ajoene, an antifungal
- Arctigenin, a lignan with anti-cancer properties
- Glabridin acid, which can prevent DNA damage caused by oxidation

Rutgers University researchers were able to isolate a particular molecule from licorice root called ß-hydroxy-DHP (BHP). BHP has the ability to stop breast and prostate cancer tumor cells while leaving healthy cells unaffected. Additionally, licorice has proven to be a powerful immune system regulator. Two compounds in licorice, Isoliquiritigenin and Naringenin, were found to promote T cell production. Another compound, Glycyrrhetinic acid, was found to protect the liver against the harmful effects of cyclophosphamide (CP), a common chemo drug.

However, we do advise patients to stop eating black licorice candy as its high sugar content can potentially raise insulin and IGF-1, which are not favorable for cancer prevention.

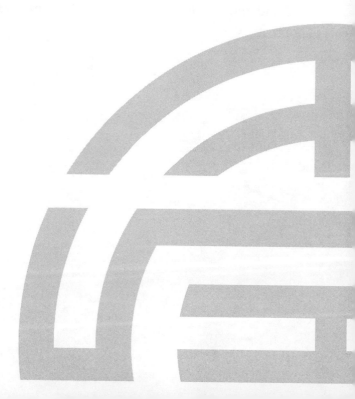

Cat's Claw Inhibits Proliferation of Leukemia Cells

Found in South America and Asia, cat's claw got its name from the claw-shaped thorns on its vine. It has been used in Chinese medicine to:

- Relax muscles
- Reduce fever-induced seizures
- Settle stomach disorders
- Enhance immune function

Studies on its alkaloids back its positive effects. In lab tests, cat's claw was shown to have anticancer effects against several cancers, as well as stimulating red and white blood cell production. Research published in the British Journal of Haematology discovered five alkaloids from cat's claw inhibited human lymphoblastic leukemia T cells. The most potent alkaloids, pteropodine (A2) and uncarine F (A4), encouraged leukemia cells to undergo apoptosis.

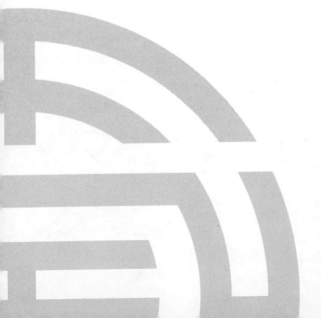

Artemisinin May Be a Therapeutic Alternative in Highly Aggressive Cancers

In 2015, the Nobel Prize in Medicine went to Tu Youyou, a Chinese scientist who discovered the active compound in the herb Artemisia. Also known as sweet wormwood or Qing Hao, the herb has 1,700 years of documented use in Chinese medicine. It is commonly used in the treatment of malaria and febrile disorders. However, it also possesses potent anticancer properties.

In a review of 127 papers published in the Annals of Medical and Health Sciences Research on the anti-cancer effects of artemisinin, researchers stated, "artemisinin compounds may be a therapeutic alternative in highly aggressive cancers with rapid dissemination, without developing drug resistance." It was found that artemisinin also exhibited synergism with other anticancer drugs with no increased toxicity toward normal cells.

The Karolinska Institute held a question-and-answer session after the announcement. There, one of the panelists praised not just the quality of Tu's scientific research, but also the value of recorded empirical experience in the long history of Chinese medicine.

Coptidis May Have a Positive Impact on Liver, Breast, and Colon Cancer Cells

The Chinese herb Huang Lian, or Coptidis, has powerful effects on cancer cells. According to a study published in Oncology Reports, one of the alkaloids from Coptidis, berberine, has been found to stimulate cell death in liver cancer cells. Berberine may interrupt liver cancer cells from dividing, thereby prohibiting cell proliferation. Another study published in Carcinogenesis showed Coptidis' effect on human breast cancer cells. An extract of Coptidis was able to inhibit breast cancer cell proliferation by increasing anticancer proteins, such as cytokines, in the body.

Other studies applied coptisine, another alkaloid from Coptidis, to colon cancer cells. One study found it to have exceptional cytotoxic activities against a specific colon cancer by inducing cell cycle arrest and it increased apoptosis. This and other studies suggest that Coptidis may have a positive impact on liver, breast, and colon cancer cells.

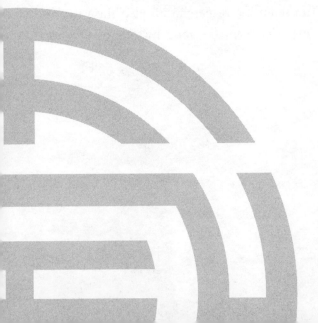

Cancer Inhibiting and Immune Bolstering Properties of the Two Sophora

Two important herbs used in Chinese medicine for cancer are Sophora flavescens (ku shen) and Sophora subprostrata (shan dou gen). Both of these herbs contain matrine and oxymatrine, alkaloids that show cytotoxic activity in lab tests and antitumor activity in humans. Oxymatrine itself has been estimated to be 7.8 times more potent than the chemo agent mitomycin C in its tumor inhibiting effects, all without suppressing the immune system. Specifically, ku shen has also been found to increase white blood cells and promote immune responses.

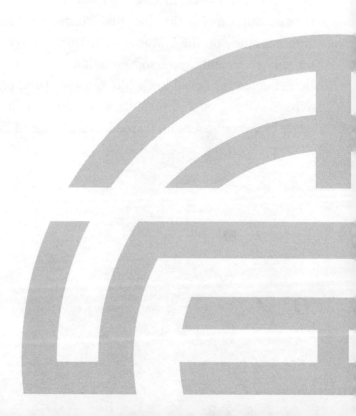

Maitake Reduces Tumor
Recurrence Rate for Bladder Cancer

Maitake mushroom, or zhu ling in Chinese, has been eaten as food in China and Japan for thousands of years. It is also an important herb used in Chinese medicine for kidney and bladder conditions. Maitake contains a wide array of bioactive molecules that stimulate natural killer (NK) cell activity in cancer patients. The mushroom has also shown promise in blocking tumor growth and activating cell death in breast cancer, lung cancer, and myelodysplastic syndromes (MDS).

One study measured tumor recurrence rates in post-surgery patients with bladder cancer. It found that when a patient underwent conventional treatment alone their cancer recurrence rate was 65%. Compared to this, patients who had the additional maitake supplementation had their recurrence rate fall to 33%. Another study on the immune bolstering action of maitake was for cancer patients receiving radiation. Those receiving radiation alone experienced low white blood cell and platelet counts. Whereas the group of patients who added maitake had their white blood cell count increased by an average of 50%.

This Root Is an Angel When It Comes to Blood Building

Angelica sinensis root, or Dang gui, has been treasured in Chinese medicine for its blood building, activating, and vitality restoring properties. It is often an indispensable culinary ingredient in chicken soup for post-surgical recovery, as well as an essential herb for women's health. Studies have confirmed that compounds in Angelica can restore bone marrow activity and help produce blood cells. It is a Fu Zheng herb, often used during chemotherapy, radiation, and post-surgery. Angelica also has anti-cancer properties.

A study published in Clinical Cancer Research determined the anti-tumor effects of Angelica on malignant brain tumors. The researchers found that Angelica had the ability to "[suppress] growth of malignant brain tumor cells without cytotoxicity to fibroblasts." This is done by a carbohydrate named APS-1d. It was also discovered to induce apoptosis of cervical cancer (HeLa cells). Continued studies are ongoing.

Massage and Bodywork Produce More Than Feel-Good Results

Who doesn't like a good massage, especially after a long week or a tension-filled day? While it's common knowledge that massage or bodywork can help relieve muscle pain, it is less known that it can actually strengthen against infection. A study published in the Journal of Anesthesia showed that leg massage significantly increased immunoglobulin proteins by 35%. In other words, massage bolsters your antibodies and immune system.

Massage and bodywork can vastly improve the quality of life for metastatic cancer patients. A study published in the Journal of Integrative and Complementary Medicine showed that providing bodywork at home for patients with advanced cancer had beneficial effects. These benefits included reductions in pain and anxiety, while enhancing the quality of life and sleep. Other studies showed that patients undergoing radiation therapy had an immediate reduction in anxiety after a massage.

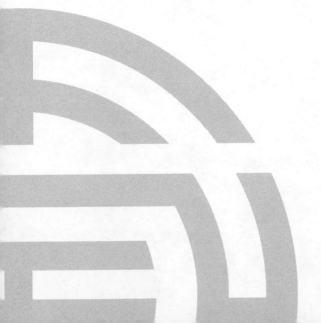

Detoxification Through Sweat Found Effective for Ridding BPA Accumulation

Bisphenol A (BPA) has been associated with an increased risk of cancer, particularly breast and prostate. That's why eliminating toxic chemicals from the body in the fastest way is vital. Researchers from the University of Alberta, Canada, conducted a study on the body's mechanisms for eliminating toxic contaminants from itself. They discovered that more BPA was found in the sweat of subjects than in their blood and urine. The findings concluded that monitoring through blood and urine testing may be miscalculating the toxic load on the body, and that sweat testing may be an additional tool for BPA monitoring. In addition, induced sweating appears to be a clinically useful tool for releasing BPA through the skin in order to eliminate this toxin from the body.

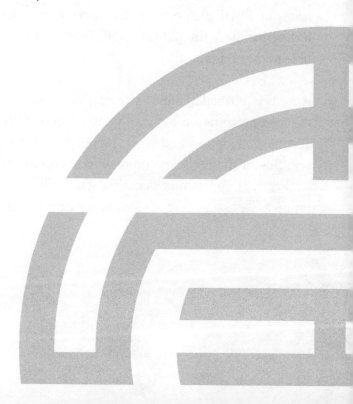

Flame Retardant Doubled Risks of Thyroid Cancer

Polybrominated diphenyl ethers (PBDEs) have been linked to thyroid cancer. They are used as flame retardants in everyday items, such as:

- Building materials
- Electronics
- Furnishings
- Cars
- Airplanes
- Plastics
- Mattresses
- Sleep wear

Researchers found that people living in homes exposed to high levels of PBDE flame retardants were at an increased risk of having papillary thyroid cancer. Children are especially susceptible to these chemicals.

A study published in Biomed Research International showed that induced perspiration helped the excretion of PBDE chemicals. Testing both blood and perspiration provides a better understanding of the body's accumulation of these carcinogens. This study gives important evidence for standardized induced perspiration as a possible way of eliminating PBDE from the body.

Sweating Is Therapeutic in Eliminating Heavy Metals

Exposure and accumulation of heavy metals such as arsenic, cadmium, lead, and mercury has been associated with degenerative neurological diseases and cancer. In conventional medicine, there is a lack of accurate testing and therapeutic intervention for this. A review of 24 studies on arsenic, cadmium, lead, and mercury detection in sweat was published in the Journal of Environmental and Public Health. These studies showed higher levels of toxic metals in sweat than in blood or urine, indicating that sweating deserves consideration for toxic element detoxification. Sweating can be induced through vigorous exercise and saunas.

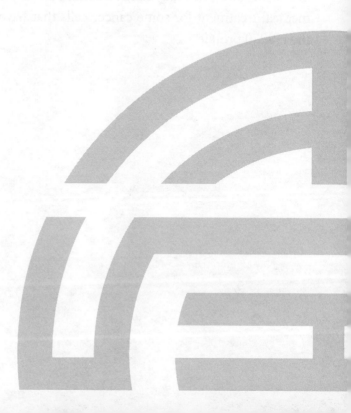

Far-Infrared Heat Found Effective in Suppressing Certain Cancers

Infrared light (IR) is the part of the light spectrum with wavelengths just longer than red. Like ultraviolet light, IR light is invisible to the naked eye but we can feel it as heat. We can also see it with the aid of technology, like night vision goggles. Far infrared (FIR) is the longest wavelength of infrared light and many studies have found that FIR possesses therapeutic properties. Now, a study shows that FIR may inhibit cancer cell proliferation.

Research published in the journal Medical Oncology found that far infrared suppressed the proliferation of some cancer cells. These cancer cells had low levels of heat shock protein 70A (HSP70), a protein which protects cancer cells from high heat exposure. The study indicates that FIR may be an effective medical treatment for some cancer cells that have low levels of the HSP70 protein.

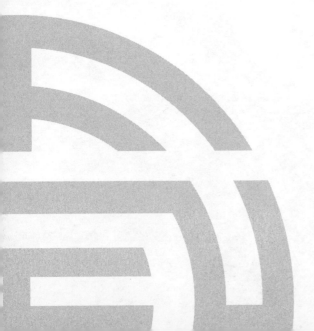

Hyperthermia May Be a Viable Adjuvant Therapy for Cancer

Hyperthermia is a type of treatment in which body tissue is exposed to high temperatures up to 113°F. Research has shown that high temperatures can damage and kill cancer cells, usually with minimal injury to normal tissues.

Hyperthermia is almost always used with other forms of cancer therapy, such as radiation therapy and chemotherapy. This is because it may make some cancer cells more sensitive to radiation or destroy other cancer cells that radiation cannot damage. Numerous clinical trials have studied hyperthermia in combination with radiation therapy and/or chemotherapy on cancers of the:

- Head
- Neck
- Brain
- Lung
- Esophagus
- Breast
- Bladder
- Rectum
- Liver
- Appendix
- Cervix
- Peritoneal lining (mesothelioma)
- Sarcoma
- Melanoma

Many of these have shown a significant reduction in tumor size when hyperthermia is combined with other treatments. Discuss with your doctor about incorporating this therapy into your current treatment protocol.

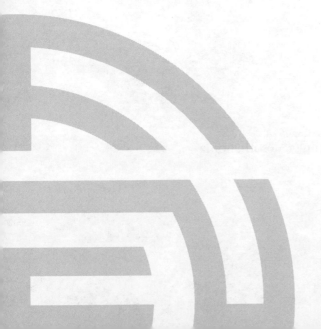

Hyperthermia Improved the Outcome for Advanced Pancreatic Cancer

Advanced pancreatic cancer patients show poor prognosis, therefore starting a treatment plan to improve their quality of life is of the utmost importance. A study published in the journal Oncology Letters showed prolonged survival rates by combining hyperthermia with chemotherapy and radiation for patients with inoperable pancreatic cancer. Researchers showed that using hyperthermia along with gemcitabine hydrochloride (a standard chemo agent for pancreatic cancer) was a safe and effective treatment modality that should be recommended to pancreatic patients.

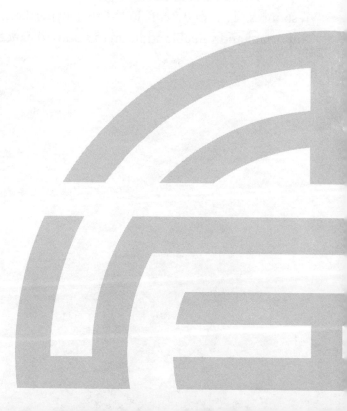

German Researchers Advocate Inclusion of Hyperthermia in Standard Cancer Care

The use of heat therapy to treat various diseases, including cancer, can be traced back to the Victorian era. The first published study was in 1866 by a German surgeon, Carl D. W. Busch (1826-1881). Currently, the use of hyperthermia as an adjuvant treatment in cancer care is applied in Asia and Europe. A study published in Frontiers in Oncology concluded that using hyperthermia to enhance the effect of radiation, chemotherapeutic agents, and immunotherapy is credible.

Other research has shown that hyperthermia may trigger increased oxygenation of tissues and cells, as well as hindering the repair mechanisms of cancer cells. Moreover, there is evidence of hyperthermia causing immune stimulation and aiding immune responses. The study concluded that hyperthermia can be an important and valuable addition to standard cancer care.

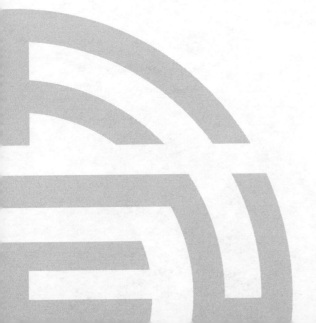

Chapter 10: Don't Be a Victim of Your Genetics

Today is a new day. Don't let your history interfere with your destiny! Let today be the day you stop being a victim of your circumstances and start taking action towards the life you want. You have the power and the time to shape your life. Break free from the poisonous victim mentality and embrace the truth of your greatness. You were not meant for a mundane or mediocre life!
— Steve Maraboli

I met Gretchen when she was 38. That was nearly 20 years ago. She had come to me with one specific purpose: not to become a victim of her own genetics.

Gretchen came from a family of four sisters and she was the youngest. Her mother and grandmother both had breast cancer at age 46 and 42, respectively. Of the three older sisters, Mary, the eldest, had breast cancer at 47. She had her stage one cancerous lump removed and underwent radiation afterwards. Elizabeth, the second oldest, was diagnosed with breast cancer at 43, had recurrence at 45, and ended up with a radical double mastectomy. Her third sister, Sheila, wasn't so lucky. She died of advanced metastatic breast cancer at age 44. It turned out all the women in her family carried the BRCA gene mutation, which made them highly susceptible to breast, ovarian, and uterine cancers.

Gretchen witnessed all the women in her family fall prey, one by one, to the ravages of breast cancer. And she was determined to not let it happen to her. She decided against undergoing prophylactic mastectomy and hysterectomy. Instead, Gretchen researched medical literature in search of cancer prevention. Her research provided her with an understanding of epigenetics, the scientific discovery that gene expression can be modified through diet, lifestyle, stress management, and even one's thoughts.

During our initial visits, I put Gretchen through a complete Chinese medicine examination and on a diet that was based on the principles of Chinese medicine. I encouraged her to change her diet towards a plant-based one filled with organics, leafy produce, brown rice, beans, legumes, and especially soy and black beans. I also discouraged all animal products except wild caught fish and organic, free range eggs. I also advised Gretchen to reduce stress in her life and take up qi gong and meditation.

Chinese Nutrition:
The Power of Food as Medicine

A high fiber, low fat, moderate protein diet is generally considered good for health. Nonetheless, recent diet trends have leaned towards high protein, high fat, and low carbohydrate diets like the ones advocated by Paleo, Ketogenic, Atkins, and others. Ultimately, there is no one-size-fits-all diet, this is why Chinese medicine has long advocated a personalized approach to diet and nutrition that is tailored to each person's constitutional and medical needs. This is especially true when it comes to diet and nutrition during cancer treatment and afterwards for preventive purposes.

Studies over the last ten years show strong links between cancer and a diet high in fat, sugar, burnt foods, commercially pickled foods, and processed foods with preservatives like nitrites, pesticides, and herbicides. The knowledge of functional foods and understanding their therapeutic properties has taught us about phytochemicals in plants that possess anti-cancer properties. Cruciferous vegetables such as broccoli, cauliflower, cabbage, and Brussels sprouts are rich in indole-3-carbinol and sulforaphane. These two particular compounds have been studied extensively. Indole-3-carbinol is a powerful anti-estrogen compound that counters cancerous growth in estrogen-sensitive cells like the breasts, colon, and prostate.

Conventional wisdom agrees that a diet that's low fat, moderate in protein, and high in both soluble and insoluble fiber is the best weapon against cancer and degenerative diseases. Yet people who have adhered to this diet still develop cancer and other diseases. Why? No doubt genetics and other relative risks, as discussed in earlier chapters, must have played a role. Additionally, a diet needs to be tailored to one's individual needs. Some people's bodies cannot handle too much fiber, while others can tolerate more fat and protein. It is also true that high amounts of animal protein, especially red meat, can lead to higher incidence of cancer.

But what if a woman who is anemic, as in the case of my patient Linda, does not improve with vegetable sources of iron and instead does best with eating red meat and livers. Does that subject her to increased cancer risks? Not necessarily. The toxins may be eliminated by eating more insoluble fiber and chlorophyll, as well as having herbal detoxification. What is important though is that because of Linda's higher protein diet, she has better energy and body functions. Therefore, she is healthier and less likely to get sick or develop cancer.

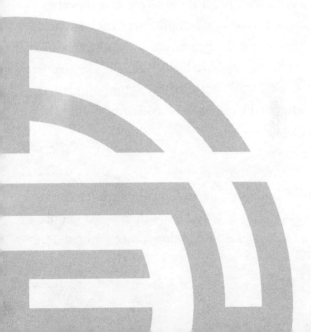

Yin and Yang Body Type

So how do you figure out what your needs are and what your diet should be? First, you must discover whether your body type is tending towards yin or yang. In other words, underdrive or overdrive, alkaline or acidic, respectively. Chinese medicine is based on the simple principle that the universe is composed of two opposite yet complementary forces. Examples of these two forces include night and day, female and male, water and fire, cold and hot, and stillness and activity.

These forces that govern nature also govern over health and disease in humans. In physics these forces are called positive and negative, strong and weak nuclear forces—all opposite yet complementary energy expressions. A doctor of Chinese medicine diagnoses the imbalance of a patient based upon patterns of biological and emotional reactions from stimuli. Symptoms and signs of cold and deficiency correspond to yin, while heat and excess correspond to yang. These patterns also relate to physiology's hypo-functions versus hyper-functions, as well as alkalinity versus acidity. Obviously, health and wellness occurs in between the two extremes of yin and yang.

The Three Health Zones

Chart 1 lists the spectrum of symptom patterns that correlate to yin and yang. A healthy constitution is reflected in the middle section called balanced optimal performance (BOP). To the left is yin, also known as underdrive or alkaline zone. To the right is yang, also known as overdrive or acidic zone.

Your body performs best in the balanced middle range, between yin and yang. If you end up to the right of the BOP, you are in the yang/acidic zone. Many studies have pointed out that acidity spurs cancerous growth, so we should move away from the side of overdrive, or yang.

What if we find ourselves to the left of BOP, in the yin zone? The yin zone represents a weakening of your body functions, in other words, under performance. This may predispose you to getting sick and a lowered metabolism. These conditions may cause slow growing fibroids, polyps, nodules, or precancerous cells that over time may turn cancerous.

Determine your body type by correlating your symptomatic tendencies in Chart 1. You may find that you have symptoms from both yin and yang zones, but see which one you fit into predominantly. You may also find out that you are already within the BOP.

The bottom-line: avoid either extreme and try to stay within the BOP.

Chart 1: the Three Health Zones

Yin Zone / ← Alkaline / Cool	Balanced Optimal Performance (BOP)	Hot / Acidic / → Yang Zone
Fatigue, pale, cold, over or underweight, loose bowel movements, not thirsty, prefers hot beverages, frequent urination, dizzy, desires physical pressure, prefers stillness	Calm disposition; normal energy, appetite, sleep, bowel habits, urination, balance of movement, and stillness; body temperature is just right	Red face, irritable, hot, thirsty, prefers cold beverages, constipated, restless, dislikes physical pressure, big appetite, dark urine, fidgety, prefers movement, insomnia

Balance Yin and Yang Body Types with Food

The key to restoring health to the BOP zone is to counter your imbalance by eating more foods from the opposite zone in order to balance out. For example, the yin body type requires more yang-warming foods, and the yang body type requires more yin-cooling foods. See Chart 2 to learn the yin-cooling and yang-warming properties of food groups. Here, we give three examples to illustrate the point.

Gretchen—Yang Body Type

For Gretchen, we determined that she was in the yang zone. She had symptoms of easy agitation, thirst for cold drinks, and constipation. Therefore, we advised that she change her diet to eat more of the food in the yin food group due to its cooling properties. In this case, Gretchen increased her consumption of vegetables, fruits, juices, teas, seaweed, algae, as well as foods in the neutral food group. She also decreased her consumption of yang foods, such as meats, sweets, and spices, until she returned to the BOP zone. Sure enough, within two weeks, she felt calmer and was no longer constipated.

Emily—Yin Body Type

Emily had determined that she was in the yin zone. This was not surprising since all she subsisted on was salads, fruits, and some occasional pasta and fish. In order to correct her imbalance and move to the BOP zone she increased her consumption of foods with warming properties. These foods included chicken, turkey, eggs, nuts and seeds, with spices such as ginger, fennel, basil, and coriander. Some foods from the neutral food group were also added, such as grains, beans, and legumes. Contrary to her worries about gaining weight, she lost the water weight she had been carrying and felt much more energetic and spry.

Danielle—Balanced Optimal Type

Danielle found herself, for the most part, pretty balanced in the BOP zone. Her challenge was to make sure she ate balanced proportions from all three food groups. In fact, she discovered that she was leaning a little too heavily into the yang foods, and as a result she was losing her patience and had recurring canker sores in her mouth. When she slightly adjusted her diet to include more yin foods, her recurring sores disappeared and she felt calmer and more relaxed.

Chart 2: Energy Properties of Foods

Yin-Cooling / Alkaline Foods	Neutral Food Group	Yang-Warming / Acidic Foods
Vegetables, veggie juice, fruits, tea, seaweed, dairy, oils, fats, fish	Grains, beans, legumes	Animal products, eggs, nuts, seeds, spices, sugar and sweets, shellfish, coffee, alcohol

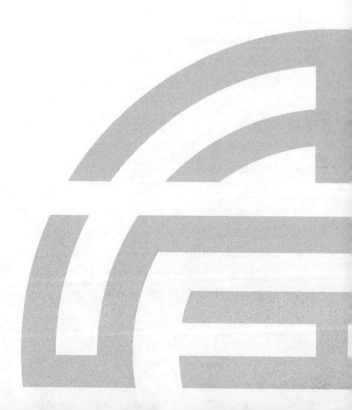

Cancer Preventing Foods

Now you will learn about additional foods that are specifically beneficial in your quest to prevent cancer. Yin alkaline foods tend to be better for cancer prevention, as they tend to discourage inflammation and cancer progression. Yin and neutral food group diets also tend to contain high fiber. This has been found to reduce inflammation, oxidative stress, and obesity, therefore lowering the risk of cancer.

Vegetables possess chlorophyll, beneficial fibers and rich sources of vitamins and minerals. Plant nutrients such as quercetin, indole-3 carbinol, and isothiocyanates increase the levels of enzymes that detoxify carcinogens in the body. Specific examples are:

- Broccoli
- Cauliflower
- Brussels sprouts
- Cabbage
- Collard greens
- Swiss chard
- Kale
- Mustard greens
- Dandelions

Further examples are:

- Mushrooms - Shitake, Maitake, Wood Ear, Button, Enoki
- Seasonal pumpkins
- Squashes - Kabocha, Butternut, Zucchini
- Cucumber
- Turnip

- Daikon radish
- Carrot
- Yam
- Sweet potato
- Asparagus

Fruits are full of fiber and antioxidant vitamins and nutrients that help prevent cancerous activities. Specific examples are:
- Tomatoes
- Citrus fruits
- Papaya
- Berries
- Apples
- Pears
- Grapes
- Cantaloupes
- Watermelon

Green and black tea are rich in plant nutrients, especially epigallocatechin, which has been found to protect against breast cancer, have antioxidants, and enhance DNA repair. In particular, women with breast cancer have a lower recurrence rate and less positive lymph nodes by drinking green tea regularly. However, due to its caffeine content, which can stimulate fibrocystic growth, we suggest limiting its consumption to one to two cups a day. This limitation does not apply to decaffeinate tea though.

Whole grains are an essential component in any cancer-prevention diet. They are filled with soluble and insoluble fibers that trap and eliminate toxins, slow down insulin release, and contain rich sources of vitamins and minerals.

Specific examples are:
- Brown rice
- Pearl barley (Job's tears)
- Millet
- Oat
- Amaranth
- Quinoa

Beans, legumes, and seeds contain plant nutrients which block harmful estrogens from binding to receptor sites in breast tissues, thereby protecting one from developing breast cancer. Specific examples are:
- Soy beans(soy milk, tofu, tempeh, miso, and bean pods)
- Black beans
- Mung beans
- Lentils
- Pumpkin seeds
- Hemp seeds
- Flax seeds

Oils contain essential fatty acids. Healthy omega 3 fatty acids are important to proper immune functions and hormonal regulation. Specific examples are:
- Olive oil
- Avocado oil
- Hemp seed oil
- Grapeseed oil
- Chia seed oil
- Flaxseed oil
- Deep sea fish oil

Spices are loaded with compounds that help block tumor forma-tion. Specific examples of powerful anti-cancer spices are:

- Ginger
- Garlic
- Onion
- Leek
- Turmeric

Try to incorporate most of the beneficial foods above into your diet, while being sure to balance your yin and yang food groups. Also try to only buy organically grown food, whenever possible.

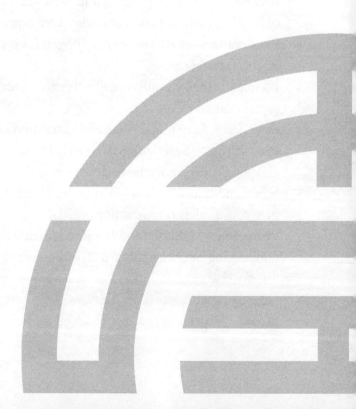

Eliminate Toxins from Your Life

Gretchen was keen on getting rid of carcinogens in her life. In her mind, applying the principles and practices of epigenetics also meant not triggering latent cancer genes with toxins. Keep in mind, however, that while carcinogens in your diet should be avoided or minimized, sometimes they may be unavoidable when you eat out, but don't worry too much. When you eat at home, you have control over what you cook, so make sure to eat more of the beneficial foods. Also, be sure to do periodic cleansing and detoxification programs to rid your body of toxins. When toxins are allowed to build-up, they may one day trigger cancer cells. Below is a list of everyday items that may be a threat to your health and wellbeing:

- Alcohol—denatures proteins and increases risk of breast, prostate, pancreatic, and liver cancers.
- Preservatives—well-known carcinogen for esophageal and stomach cancer.
- Food coloring—cumulative effects can increase risk of certain cancers.
- Deep fried, fatty foods—fats and denatured fats have been found to be a strong cause of breast cancer by elevating estrogen in the body.
- Hormone-injected meat—stimulates abnormal growths in breast and other reproductive organs.
- Processed and refined foods—nutritionally inferior and lacking in critical fiber which protects against cancer and toxic accumulation.
- Cow dairy with growth hormones—stimulates abnormal growths, especially in the breast and reproductive tissues.

- Barbequed, burnt, or blackened food—increase the risk of cancer in the digestive lining.
- Pickled food or processed meats with nitrites—part of the preservative family of chemicals that can cause cancer.
- Poultry and eggs from birds injected with growth hormones—same problem as the meats and dairy with growth hormones, can create abnormal growth in breast and reproductive tissues.
- Vegetables and fruits sprayed with pesticides and herbicides—often mimics estrogen in the body, thereby increasing risk of breast and other reproductive cancers.

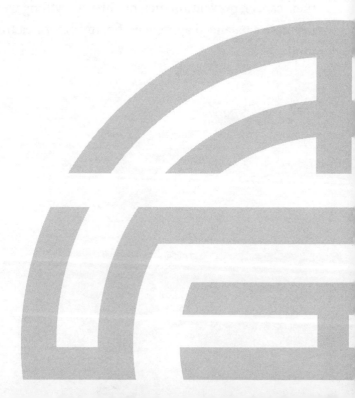

What About Soy?
Soy Protects, Rather Than Causes Breast Cancer

Gretchen was afraid of eating soy for a long time. She had been told by her breast specialist to avoid soy because it "causes breast cancer." Research tells us otherwise. Soy is probably the most researched food in the world. Well over 1,000 studies have been conducted worldwide in an attempt to discover the medical benefits of this Asian staple. A majority of the studies conclude that soy benefits heart health, due to its cholesterol lowering property. It can also have a breast cancer protective property due to its ability to bind estrogen-receptor sites, due to its plant based estrogen called genistein. This means that "bad" estrogens (like the ones from pesticides, BPA, contraceptive pills, and replacement estrogen) cannot bind to the receptor sites in the breast tissue. Clinically, we advise women to incorporate soy as a part of their cancer-prevention diet, but like everything we advocate, we promote a balanced approach of many other healthy and helpful foods.

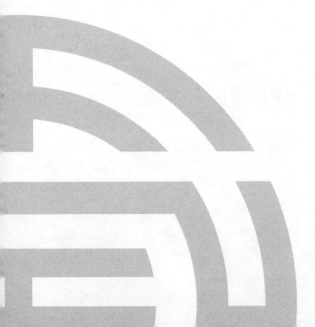

Plant-Based Eating Is Best for Both Your Health and The Environment

Most vegetarians and vegans tend to find themselves leaning towards the yin zone. This is due to their dietary tendencies of eating mostly cooling and neutral foods. A plant-based diet results in lowered incidence of most cancers according to some research studies. However, if a vegetarian is chronically in the yin zone they must make sure their functions do not decline and become anemic. This is done by supplementing with vitamin B12 and D, which are usually missing from the diets of vegetarians. So again, the key to effective disease and cancer prevention is to regularly adjust your diet in order to achieve, based on your symptom pattern, the balanced optimal performance (BOP) zone at all times.

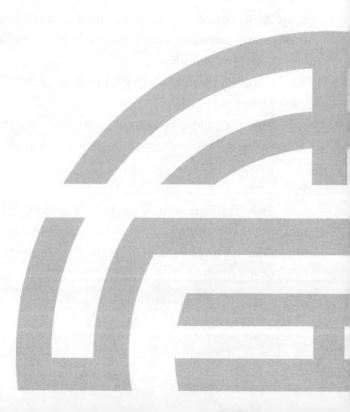

The Role of Antioxidant Supplements and Nutraceuticals

Much research has been done and more is on the way with regards to dietary supplements and nutraceuticals, and their roles as cancer-prevention agents. Nutraceuticals, derived from the words nutrition and pharmaceutical, are foods which work as medicines. The theory of free radical damage has long been proposed and recently confirmed as one of the causes of cancerous growth in the body. As free radicals are released through defective metabolism, poor diet, and environmental toxins, they damage DNA throughout the body.

As the damaged cellular DNAs reproduce, they create new cells that are also flawed. This new generation of cells can have the potential of turning into uncontrollable, cancerous cells. That is the main reason cancer prevention research has zeroed in on antioxidant nutrients, which include but are not limited to:

- Vitamin C and E
- Carotenoids like lycopene, lipoic acid, and CoQ10
- Flavonoids
- Enzymes, like glutathione peroxidase, which inhibit and "mop up" corrosive, free oxygen atoms that cause damage to cells.

Antioxidants primary function is to defend against harmful free radicals. Their secondary function includes DNA repair mechanisms. See Chapter 5 for more in depth discussion of many antioxidant nutrients.

Micronutrient Testing to Discover What You Need

Gretchen wanted to take antioxidants and other dietary supplements. But she was hesitant to blindly take the bewildering variety of products at health food stores often manned by clerks who looked in books and "prescribed" them to customers. We made it easy for her and took out the guesswork by prescribing a micronutrient blood test to determine if any deficiencies were present. It came back that she tested low for folic acid, vitamin D, Coenzyme Q10, and her ratio of omega fatty acids were not optimal. She then knew definitively, instead of guessing, what she needed to take.

Before you rush out and buy a bag full of supplements, we advocate having a micronutrient test. This can be done either through blood or urine testing, and it will determine nutrient levels. It tests for nutrients ranging from vitamins A-Z, amino acids, fatty acids, and antioxidants. Once we receive the lab test results, we can then advise our patients. First we identify food sources for the deficient nutrients, then we recommend supplements with high quality nutritional products. Remember, these are supplements and are not replacements. Getting your maximum nutrition from your diet is still our top recommendation.

Cancer Prevention as a Lifestyle

It has been 20 years since Gretchen implemented the nutritional program I recommended to her. She has enjoyed good health and so far has avoided the breast disease that seemed destined to strike her down due to her genetics. At age 58–as of the release of this book–Gretchen is eight years past her menopause and firmly believes that her diet, which now has become a lifestyle, is the single most important factor in having helped her prevent breast cancer thus far.

Many of my patients have shared similar beneficial experiences to Gretchen's. Diet and nutrition is but one of a number of methods presented in this book to lower one's risk of cancer, however it is a powerful one. By combining natural principles of balance, optimal health with Chinese medicine's dietetic traditions, and scientific investigation of clinical nutrition and food functions, everyone shall have the knowledge and opportunity to implement a sound diet and nutrition for cancer prevention.

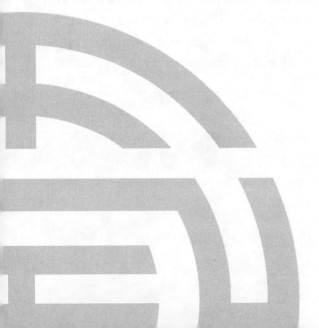

Chapter 11: Cancer Journeys — Patients' Experience with Integrative Cancer Care and Prevention

It is often in the darkest skies that we see the brightest stars.
—*Richard Paul Evans*

We asked a few of our patients to share their cancer journeys with us for this book in the hopes that they can be inspirations for others facing similar challenges. When requested, we used pseudonyms for those who wanted to preserve their privacy.

My Healing Journey by Phyllis Koenig
(excerpts transcribed from an interview on the Healing Hour Show featured on Tao of Wellness' YouTube channel)

My story is actually really stupid, it started out with pure negligence. I've always been healthy and strong. In fact, I was running a business that employed many people and knew literally thousands of people. I was proud that I was working hard, being successful, and feeling strong. All this despite knowing that on my mother's side, her brother, sister, cousin, and others all died of cancer. But in my head, I thought since it skipped my mother I was fine. I never thought it would ever happen to me. When I was first diagnosed, I had a four centimeter lump in my left breast. I thought it was nothing, it moved around and since I'm very cystic, it was not a big deal. So I just kept moving forward and never stopped for a moment.

When I went to the doctor and had my mammogram, the doctor said afterwards, "Hey, do you mind waiting for a few minutes while we look at your imaging?" So I sat in a lonely chair watching everyone walk by. Twenty minutes later the doctors came out and said, "Do you mind if we take some tissue from you? It's probably nothing, but we just want to make sure." So I waited for another 20 minutes and after the biopsy I left in a sling. Eventually, 3-4 days later, I got a call on a Monday morning and the doctor said, "You'd better come down here—you are very, very sick." That was the beginning of my journey.

I went from being the strongest woman to being a hysterical woman—I was a mess! I was lucky enough to find Dr. Kristi Funk, a breast cancer surgeon. She was this beautiful, petite doctor, pregnant with triplets, and she said, "I want you to wrap your head around Chinese medicine and go see Dr. Mao at the Tao of Wellness in Santa Monica." As soon as I met Dr. Mao I knew I was going to be fine. I went through surgery, chemo, and estrogen blocking under the care of Dr. Philomena McAndrew, all the while getting acupuncture treatments from Dr. Mao and taking his herbs and supplements. That kept me alive and here I am.

It was wonderful because it was stage 4 metastatic breast cancer and I had three months to live, according to my Western medicine doctors. That was until I found Dr. Mao at the Tao of Wellness. My experience was that I didn't have to go through Western medicine alone. With Dr. Mao being versed in Western medicine too, he was an essential part of the decision-making process when it came to my integrative care for both medicines. I recently had my 11th year anniversary and even my Western doctor said, "You are so wild, we never expected you to live past one year and the fact that you made it past 10 years... we don't know what to do with you." I am grateful and happy that I can share my story so that others in similar situations may be helped by hearing it.

A Healing Story by Alicia Sky Varinaitus-Kunerth
(Reprinted from the Tao of Wellness Newsletter)

"You have a brain tumor." At age 30 and eight months pregnant with my first child, it was the last thing I expected to hear out of the doctor's mouth. I had never been sick or dizzy. Had never felt nauseous or woozy or had headaches. One day, without explanation or forewarning, I began to have grand mal seizures. Mark, my husband of two years, was the one who found me in our home office, seizing. He called 911 and I was rushed to the emergency room. A pregnancy condition called Eclampsia was first suspected, but after two brain scans, we were told that the cause of the seizures was a golf ball sized tumor in my left frontal lobe. I remember thinking, "This isn't happening. This can't be real." I was immediately admitted into the High Risk Pregnancy Ward at Encino-Tarzana Hospital, where I stayed for six weeks until the birth of our beautiful daughter, Ashlyn Pearl. Seven days later, having recovered enough from the C-section delivery, I was transferred to Cedars-Sinai Hospital for brain surgery. A wonderful surgeon, Dr. Keith Black, did an amazing job removing the tumor. Afterwards, he informed my husband that the surgery had gone "very well" and that he was confident he had "gotten everything he could see."

One week later, Mark and I were in Dr. Black's office to review the tumor biopsy results. With hopes of "please let it be nothing" floating around in our heads, we were floored by the results. The tumor was classified as a Grade IV Glioblastoma Multiforme. The doctor's exact words were, "These types of tumors are incurable…" My first thought was, "I won't see my daughter take her first steps." Sorrow, grief, heartbreak, despair – it's hard to accurately describe what we were feeling. To their ultimate credit, the doctors handling my case were always extremely positive and quick to remind us that although the tumor wasn't curable, it was highly treatable. I was young, in good health, and a woman – three factors that put me way ahead of the norm in terms of life expectancy. The ordered course of treatment: seven weeks of daily radiation done concurrently with monthly oral chemotherapy.

Even though I knew that the radiation and chemotherapy would be hard, I was extremely surprised at how much the treatments drained me. The medications I was taking made it unsafe to nurse my daughter and they also made me too tired to stay awake through a single bottle-feeding. I was spending most of my days knocked out in bed just trying to keep down chicken broth and crackers. And, due to the intense radiation treatments, I was losing my hair. I still remember the day I was in the shower and chunks of my hair just began falling out. I didn't even have to pull. That was the day it hit me, "I'm truly sick." I was weak, exhausted, and overcome by depression. Despite all the books I read about positive mind over matter, I couldn't find the energy or the will to even begin to battle the cancer.

The Western Medicine approach to my disease was slowly obliterating my life. It would take something powerful to turn my life around. That was when a friend told me about the Tao of Wellness.

My friend was being treated by Dr. Mao for an especially severe case of lymphoma. I will readily admit I was a skeptic of Eastern medicine, including acupuncture. I didn't see how small pins poked into the skin could amount to anything substantial. So, I don't know exactly what it was – perhaps my friend's copious enthusiasm or perhaps I was just too tired to protest – but I am so enormously grateful I agreed to meet with Dr. Mao.

Dr. Mao prescribed a combination of a healthy diet, herbs, and acupuncture which helped tremendously (and immediately) with my never-ending fatigue and nausea. I was able to keep food down, which meant I started to gain weight, which in turn helped me grow physically and emotionally stronger. I learned to meditate, which cleared my mind for powerful healing suggestions. I found I was no longer held hostage by the fear of dying. I couldn't necessarily quantify my positive reaction to the treatment in physical, easy to see terms, but I felt better on the inside. And that made all the difference in the world.

About three months after I started with Dr. Mao, I had a follow-up exam with my radiation oncologist. I thought that after the radiation treatments were completed my hair would return. The hair not affected by the treatments had started to grow, but I still had a very large, noticeable bald spot on the left side of my head. It was funny how much I resembled my infant daughter – both of us had a ring of hair around the base of our skull, but the top of our heads were smooth. During the exam, I asked when I should expect my hair to return. She paused, I think cautious of my fragile emotional state, and said gently, "The radiation levels your tumor required were very intense. The hair follicles in that area are most likely destroyed."

Looking back, I should have hit my knees in thankfulness for the technology that could burn away any remnants of cancer cells that surgery had left behind, but in truth I was devastated. It's hard to gauge the progress of your healing unless you can look at yourself and see actual positive changes. Without my hair, I looked sick. Since I looked sick, I felt sick. My doctor was saying my hair would never grow back. Who was I to dispute her educated assessment?

Later that day, Dr. Mao walked into the treatment room to find me sitting on the table, weeping. I could barely speak, I was crying so hard. Upon hearing what my doctor had told me he said, "You must never listen to doctors – not even me. Every single person is different. No one can tell you what your body will and will not do." He then brought in a small bottle of herbal liquid and told me, "Scrub this on your head with a toothbrush twice a day. It will make your hair sprout." I took the liquid home and did what Dr. Mao had told me to do. About three weeks later I couldn't believe my eyes. There were actual "sprouts." My hair was growing back! About six months later I returned to the oncologist that had deemed my head a barren wasteland and she was stunned. She even wondered out loud (jokingly, let's hope) if she had administered the correct dosage of radiation. Six months after that I had my first real full-head-of-hair haircut. That was a great day.

Dr. Mao's advice not to take everything a doctor says to heart was profound. And I truly believe the brown herbal formula he prescribed regenerated my hair follicles. But it was a simple story he told that day that gave me the inspiration to start reliving my life. He told me to be happy because I looked like a Buddhist monk. I wasn't in a place where I could joke about my baldness, but Dr. Mao insisted he wasn't teasing. He asked, "Do you know why Buddhist monks shave the top of their heads?" I did not. He told me, "It makes them closer to God."

That's what I had come to Dr. Mao to hear. Instantly, all my sadness and fear about being bald for the rest of my life melted away. It was what I had been praying for all along. I needed to hear that God was by my side, battling my disease with me. I accepted, truly for the first time, God's will instead of my own.

In July of this year, I will be two years cancer free. I believe I am cured. If ever an MRI shows any tumor regrowth, I feel confident I will beat it. And if I don't and it is my turn to pass from this life, I will not fear the unknown. I will embrace it. Thanks, in large part, to Dr. Mao.

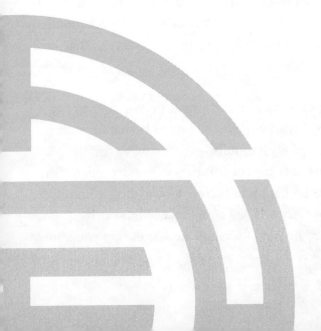

Sandra M.

I was diagnosed with breast cancer in September, 2016. My diagnosis was that I had a very "good" curable kind, but would need to undergo chemo, radiation, and surgeries—which did not sound like the "good" kind to me at all.

Tao of Wellness was immediately recommended to me by people I knew who were undergoing or had undergone the same thing. For me, the chemotherapy was incredibly difficult, but acupuncture, mainly under Frances Lam's care, was incredibly helpful and healing. My sessions were specifically scheduled between chemotherapy treatments, along with supportive herbs to boost my immune system and lessen my side effects, especially the nausea.

Frances was incredibly helpful with food recommendations and suggestions for things I could tolerate at the most difficult times. I was emotionally supported by Frances as well, who was always encouraging during this difficult journey.

I am now two years away from that diagnosis and all healed! I am cured and strong and vibrant and I still get acupuncture on a regular basis, and I am forever grateful to Frances and the staff at the Tao of Wellness for their service to me.

Carol B.

I have been a patient of Dr. Mao's since my breast surgeon referred me to him in the spring of 2011, after I received my initial stage 2/3 breast cancer diagnosis. I'll never forget, my husband and I were sitting in his office and before the first tear had fallen from my eyes he had already offered me a tissue.

I think I was sharing how one of my dreams in life is to someday be a grandmother, having never known my own, although as a mom of two young girls at the time, I wasn't in a rush - just hoping to be blessed with the time to see that dream become reality. He said, "You'll be a great grandma." His kind, positive encouragement and extensive knowledge of health, wellness, and healing continues to be a crucial part of my care.

During chemo, when I experienced neuropathy, he treated it with acupuncture and saw me before my next infusion which success-fully prevented it from occurring again. The day of my bilateral mastectomy, Dr. Mao's associate treated me with acupuncture while I was recovering from surgery to help me detox from the anesthesia and get my "qi" flowing.

Dr. Mao's customized Chinese teas and supplements help keep my immune system strong during various cancer treatments and when facing other health challenges; from allergy season sinus headaches to altitude sickness on ski trips, and ear infections from my oceanic adventures in scuba diving and swimming with dolphins.

Dr. Mao likes to joke that I may be a little too active sometimes and need my rest. Listening to his Taoist meditation series has helped me to learn also enjoy slowing down, and watching his Qi Gong for Cancer DVD has been a revelation since my metastatic breast cancer diagnosis in the fall of 2017.

My last scans were stable to improved. I am planning to study Qi Gong/Infinchi Energy Healing at Yo San University, a school founded by Dr. Mao and his brother, this January. I hope to be able to help others with cancer feel the amazing restorative power and peaceful bliss qi gong brings to me each time I practice it. Thank you Dr. Mao for everything you do to help me and so many others.

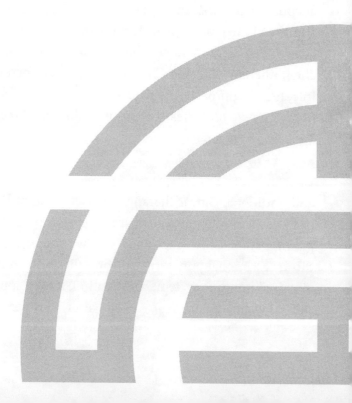

Our Son's Journey with Leukemia

When our son, James B., was diagnosed at 11 months of age with high-risk infantile leukemia, our family was devastated. We spent months in the hospital for treatment, and the side effects of the chemo combined with multiple life-threatening infections nearly took his life a number of times. James lost 25% of his body weight in a matter of weeks and suffered numerous developmental setbacks. Combined with intense pain, he was suffering immeasurably.

As a childhood cancer survivor myself, I knew the importance of combining a holistic and integrative approach to James' traditional Western medicine treatment. Once James was stable, we immediately sought the help and support of Dr. Mao and his team at Tao of Wellness to support James' cancer treatment with acupuncture, herbs, and Eastern medicine. We also worked with additional integrative providers for nutritional/supplement and cannabis related therapy. The combination of the traditional chemotherapy with the Chinese herbs, acupuncture, and other integrative approaches provided a synergy and strengthening of treatment for James that he wouldn't have received with a Western approach alone.

Over the course of James' two and a half years of chemotherapy and traditional cancer therapy, we visited Tao of Wellness twice per week and integrated their treatments as part of our wellness plan for him. James continued to have some side effects from the drugs, lumbar punctures, and anesthesia, including a severely impaired immune system, constipation, loss of appetite, nausea, skin problems, poor sleep, etc. However, they were significantly minimized due to his acupuncture and integrative therapy.

From the first acupuncture treatment, we immediately began to see a positive difference in James. By using the acupuncture treatments combined with herbal formulas, tuina massage, and other integrative approaches, James steadily began to gain weight, get stronger, recover faster from chemotherapy, sleep better, and have a brighter disposition in general. We were able to manage and greatly minimize his nausea, his insomnia, and his pain so that he could get a foothold in his recovery and not only endure but thrive during the remaining journey of his chemotherapy treatment.

James finished his last chemo treatment at the end of October 2018, and he remains in remission from his cancer. At this point, he has very few lasting side effects from the chemo, surgeries, and procedures, and we credit that to acupuncture, Eastern medicine, cannabis, and other integrative therapies. Although he still has some catching up to do to fully reach his peer level, he is living the life of a normal child. We plan to continue utilizing Eastern medicine to keep James strong, healthy, and in remission. In addition to acupuncture and tuina massage, we have found that James really enjoys cupping and bodywork as well. He enjoys taking his herbal preparations and accepts the acupuncture needles like a champion. James is a true warrior in body and a beacon of light in spirit.

We truly believe James' healing success is due to our integrative approach. We are dedicated to keeping him well, and we will always rely upon Eastern and integrative approaches to complement Western medicine in order to keep his body, mind, and spirit balanced and healthy.

Jerry S.

I have been coming to Tao of Wellness since 2012 and working with Frances Lam since about 2014. I have been getting acupuncture since 2005, initially in the Bay Area. First, I started treatments along with my wife to improve our chances of getting pregnant. We were fortunate to have 2 children with the help of acupuncture and Chinese herbs.

After our second child was born in 2011, I continued with acupuncture as a general "maintenance" measure that I feel helped me reduce stress and maintain more of an emotional equilibrium. I felt acupuncture and Chinese herbs were an integral part of a holistic health regimen that included diet and exercise. Then, in early 2017, I was diagnosed with colon cancer.

I embarked on what was frankly a terrifying journey of surgery, radiation, and chemotherapy that consumed most of that year. As I headed into 2018, with the help of Frances and another integrative care specialist, I have "doubled down" on the holistic approach: extending my prior routine of acupuncture and Chinese herbs to a stricter diet which meant no red meat, no cured meat, drastically reduced sugar and refined carbs, more vegetables, and antioxidant-rich fruits.

I also embarked on more frequent cardio exercise 3 times per week, weight training twice per week, 9 holes of golf, flexibility and stretching every morning, as well as key supplements of daily vitamins, omega-3 fatty acids, medicinal mushroom supplements, resveratrol, curcumin, green tea extract, among others and occasional meditation.

While I recently got a second clean scan, I'm not sure what the future holds. Yet, I cannot stress enough the psychic benefit and sense of empowerment that comes from this more holistic, integrative approach. Frances has been a critical and key proponent of this approach to actively manage my condition. I continue to be forever grateful for her counsel and friendship.

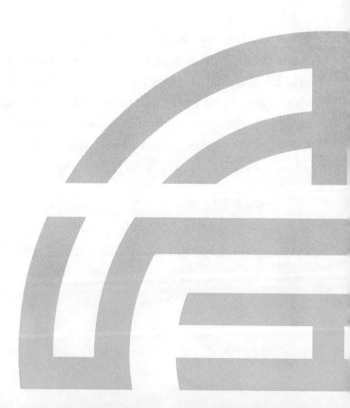

My Spiritual Journey Through Cancer by Charlene Sato

My first episode of breast cancer was at the age of 57. It was Stage 1, estrogen positive and curable. I had minor surgery and 33 radiation therapy treatments. Then, nine years later during a routine mammogram, the radiologist saw a shadow but the location was unclear. There was no indication of a tumor or calcification around the breast area. I immediately requested an ultrasound and biopsy, because I knew that if it was cancer there would be other tests and there would be decisions to be made.

The shadow was one lymph node within the left axilla, the size was 1.17cm. The biopsy report indicated occult breast cancer, Stage 2, triple negative, which is a very aggressive type of breast cancer. When I heard the news from my breast surgeon it was hard to accept.

There had not been any breast cancer in my family; I ate healthy foods (mainly plant based), taught tai chi/chi gong, did daily meditation, went to the gym, never smoked, drank a glass of alcohol four times a year, and slept 8 to 9 hours a night. My oncologist and other doctors did not know why I had a new cancer on the other breast. Fortunately, I was assured that the new cancer was curable, because of the early detection.

This second time around, I would have to receive chemotherapy, surgery, and radiation. The thought of chemotherapy made me anxious, afraid, and sad. The thought of losing all my hair, feeling nausea, extreme fatigue, losing weight, etc. was not appealing.

I had to ask myself, why do I have cancer again? This second time, it was a big spiritual awakening. When I was diagnosed with the occult breast cancer, my immediate thought was; I have unfinished business on this earth. Before I leave my body, I want to become more spiritually evolved to help others. However, I need to first learn self-care and self-compassion and to be mindful before I could practice compassion towards others.

Through this spiritual journey of cancer, I am learning to have positive thoughts for myself, which is the beginning of self-care. I was brought up thinking what I did was important but not who I am. All my life, I was striving and always thinking what I did was the key to be accepted and loved by others. But now I know that who I am is enough even with all my imperfections.

The mind is very powerful and when one does not have positive thoughts constantly about oneself, it can affect one's spirit and body. As human beings, we are an integration of mind, body, and spirit. When our minds are calm and relaxed then our bodies are able to be less tense and our muscles can relax.

With acupuncture treatments during chemotherapy, my body was able to relax and at the same time feel energized. I received tremendous energetic support from Dr. Mao's acupuncture treatment. I never would have gotten through, especially towards the end of the chemo sessions, if I had not received those treatments with Dr. Mao.

Both cancer episodes I was supported by dedicated doctors at the Tao of Wellness, especially by Dr. Mao and his brother Dr. Daoshing Ni, who are exceptionally knowledgeable, dedicated, and compassionate doctors, and who are also healers.

I am lucky to be given a third chance at LIFE with the support of wonderful doctors who practice Eastern and Western medicine to eradicate the disease of cancer. As a Shinnyo en Buddhist practitioner, I received spiritual support and guidance to be grateful every moment, to find JOY in helping others, and most importantly to BELIEVE in myself. Also, I am learning to LOVE and ACCEPT myself for who I am. I have FAITH in the higher spirit guiding me towards the light during the darkest moments through the journey of cancer.

Hopefully, in the future no one will suffer or die from cancer. Until then, acupuncture, tai chi and chi gong daily exercise, meditation practice, eating well, getting plenty of sleep, and having positive thoughts and gratitude are tools that I have found to stay healthy, happy, and strong.

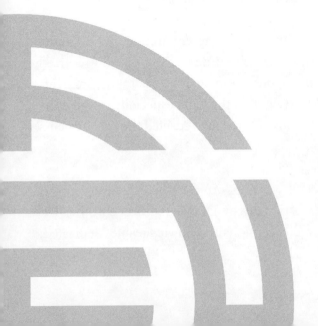

Gina W.

Receiving a diagnosis of cancer, even a slow-moving one like chronic lymphocytic leukemia, is a very frightening experience. I felt perfectly fine, had worked hard throughout my life to stay in shape and eat right, and suddenly felt like my body and my DNA had turned on me for no reason.

A friend of mine suggested that I see Dr. Mao at Tao of Wellness as Traditional Chinese Medicine had helped him with several health issues he was facing. I was interested, but initially skeptical--my grandfather had been an M.D. and I had been raised to view other forms of medicine with a bit of suspicion. It was only when an M.D. I was seeing told me she was taking a sabbatical to study alternative medicine that I realized I was limiting my thinking for no good reason.

From the first moment I met with Dr. Mao and his associate Frances Lam, I sensed that I was in capable, experienced hands. After meeting with me, they prescribed a week-long cleansing diet, gave me a list of foods with cancer-fighting properties, and began a weekly schedule of acupuncture treatment combined with daily herbs.

After several weeks I began to notice that I was losing weight in a healthy way and that my overall energy and vitality was increasing. The acupuncture treatments are very pleasant and I began to look forward to them for their nurturing and comforting properties. After three months under their care, I went to see my M.D. who informed me that my blood numbers had all improved.

This was very welcome news indeed, and I look forward to continuing my treatments with Dr. Mao and Frances, delaying the time that I might require chemotherapy or other treatments, perhaps even for the rest of a long and healthy life.

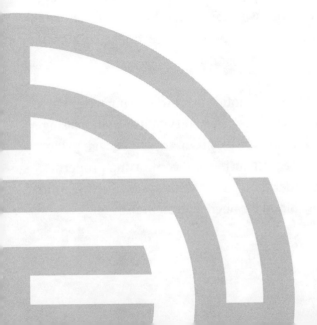

Howard Epstein

Summary: A unique combination of mostly Traditional Chinese Medicine (TCM) herbal supplements and Off-Label prescription drugs slowed down the progression of my "Always Fatal" CLL (chronic lymphocytic leukemia). Finally, after about 10 years with such treatments, a well targeted "Big Pharma" drug was released. When added to my other protocol, it reversed my disease. 4 years after adding Ibrutinib, my tumor load is down about 97%. My CLL is now controlled but not yet "cured".

During my first few years with CLL, I followed a diet recommended by Dr. Mao Shing Ni, a 38th generation doctor of Chinese medicine near Los Angeles. I also regularly brewed tea that Dr. Mao specially formulated for me. I lived in the San Jose area at the time.

After moving to Portland, Oregon, I found and added to my team an Integrative Medicine Cancer Specialist in Ashland, Oregon, Donnie Yance, who was highly trusted by my Oncologist in Portland. In addition to trusting my herbal protocol, Dr. Daniel Gruenberg also accepted advice from Yance on the "Western" medicine and dosages Yance recommended. Dr. Gruenberg often thanks me for bringing useful "tools" to his practice and doing better than most similar patients. Sadly, such open minded oncologists are rare in this country.

Very important is the fact that I was able to bypass the standard recommendation of FCR. (chemotherapy). FCR is usually effective and extends life 2 to 4 years before almost all become ineffective. Without FCR, my form of CLL should have given me a median lifetime of about 2.5 years after my diagnosis in 2004. With it, about 5 to 6 years. I lasted 10 years before Ibrutinib was finally released. This and several other new drugs have now made CLL controllable for most.

As a person who spent 40 years doing scientific research, I am abhorred that oncologists cannot accept that 3,000 years of careful observation is scientifically valid. Medical doctors think they understand statistics, but their understanding is most shallow and most Western medical procedures are also based on tradition, rather than "evidenced" based.

My oncologist is retiring. On Monday, I saw a research oncologist, trained first in Russia, who is at our local medical school. Russian docs, I think, are not as well versed in herbal medicine as Chinese doctors. But they are less disrespectful than most MDs trained in the US. He admitted that I am doing quite well and saw no reason why he would want to change what I am doing, if he became my oncologist. He was also humble enough to say that he would have recommended against my protocol earlier. He is not so interested in studying what evidence supports my herbal protocol. I can continue with him, but my case will remain anecdotal, not something he will have anyone pursue at all in the research lab for Hematological Malignancies that he heads.

Because I continued my other protocol, including Chinese medicine, I was able to get full efficacy with a small fraction of Ibrutinib's normal dose and have not had any adverse side effects. I am happy to report that 14 years after my initial diagnosis, my tumor load is down about 97% and my CLL is now controlled.

Stephanie A.

In February 2017, I was diagnosed with a chronic form of leukemia. After consulting with The City of Hope and a private oncologist, I was told that the numbers that I was presented with didn't require that I seek immediate treatment.

When I asked my oncologist what I needed to do, he told me that I really didn't need to change anything in my lifestyle, until it was determined I needed to start treatment. My diagnosis brought extreme stress into my life and I wasn't really content to continue living my life as if nothing was going on.

A friend of mine suggested that I meet with Dr. Mao Shing Ni, who had helped her with health issues she has faced herself. Dr. Mao had an instant calming effect on me. I immediately felt not only understood, but comforted. He told me the exact opposite of what I had been told.

He advised that I needed to take a proactive approach and to change not only my lifestyle, but also my diet. He explained in detail what foods to stay away from and which anti-cancer ones to add. He also designed a combination treatment that included acupuncture, nutrition, and a formulation of Chinese herbs that I had to take every day. As a result, my numbers have stayed steady.

Dr. Mao's and Frances Lam's expertise, as well as their wisdom, understanding, and caring about how I feel, has had a profound effect on me. I have since recommended Dr. Mao to friends and family members, and he has had the same profound effect in their lives.

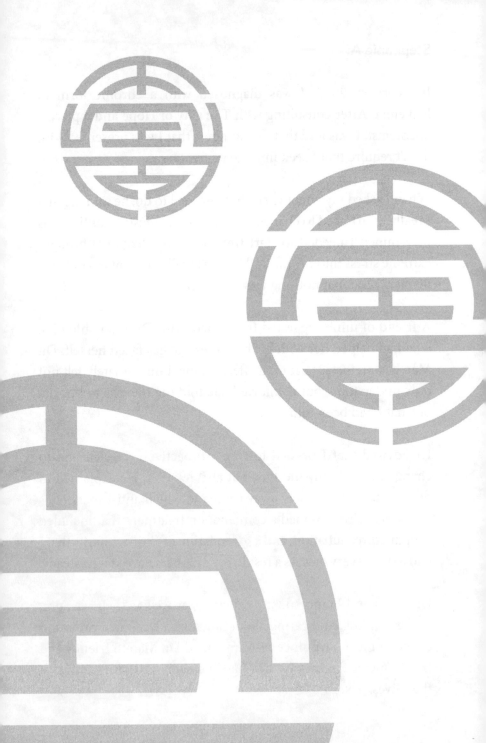

Chapter 12: Cannabis for Cancer – Fact or Fiction?

Cannabis, or ma, has been cultivated and used by the Chinese for food, clothing, paper and medicine as far back as 8,000 years ago. It was prized as both a food and medicine plant. The original text of the Shen Nong Ben Cao, or Divine Farmer's Classic of Materia Medica, ascribes the following properties to cannabis:

Ma fen benefits the five viscera by repairing strains to the five viscera, treats the seven injuries (overeating injures the spleen, rage injures the liver, dampness injuries the kidneys, cold injuries lungs, sadness injures heart, wind injures body, fear injuries will to live), breaks up blood stagnation, and cools heat; excessive consumption causes one to see ghosts and run about frantically. Regular consumption frees the spirit, elevates consciousness and lightens the body. The seed, ma zi, possesses sweet flavor and neutral property, strengthens core, benefits qi, and retards aging as elixir for immortality. It is grown in verdant valleys.

During the second century A.D., the Chinese surgeon Hua Tuo used cannabis as an anesthesia. He combined cannabis resin with wine and used it to reduce pain during surgery. The Chinese term for anesthesia, ma zui, literally means "cannabis intoxication," which shows a knowledge of the narcotic properties of cannabis as far back as Julius Cesar. The Great Encyclopedia of Chinese Medicinals states that ma fen "dispels wind, relieves pain, and settles tremors." According to this text, it is used for conditions traditionally known as "impediment patterns."

These manifest as:
- Pain
- Restricted movement
- Gout
- Withdrawal
- Mania
- Insomnia
- Panting
- Coughing

It's apparent from various Chinese medical texts spanning at least two millennia that cannabis' properties had been valued by physicians for:
- Anti-inflammatory
- Anti-seizure
- Antispasmodic
- Analgesic
- Psychoactive

Additionally, the rich omega fatty acid and antioxidant contents of hemp seeds made it highly prized as a superfood for health and anti-aging. Finally, a special feature of cannabis is how it is used as part of a formulation to achieve therapeutic synergy with multi-ingredient remedies. For example, Chinese herb-infused CBD formulas can increase terpenoid content and enhance both entourage and therapeutic effects. This is discussed more in-depth in the following pages.

Tetrahydrocannabinol (THC) is the psychoactive component of cannabis. Since the laboratory synthesis of THC in the 1970s, research has delved into the various compounds of cannabis in an attempt to better understand its therapeutic value. Many of the studies have centered on cannabidiol (CBD). However, cannabis contains hundreds of other compounds such as terpenoids, flavonoids, and essential fatty acids.

In recent years, the cancer community has been excited by research that has shown that CBD may have anti-cancer properties. For example, a preclinical study by Dr. Sean McAllister and his colleagues at the California Pacific Medical Center in San Francisco reported on how CBD destroys breast cancer cells. It does this by reducing ID-1, a gene which is implicated in several types of aggressive cancer.

In this chapter, we will attempt to provide an overview of cannabis, its therapeutic components, and the latest research findings. We will also provide questions cancer patients and caregivers should be asking and discussing with both their oncologist and cannabis providers when it comes to incorporating it into their overall cancer treatment plan.

Conduit Between Brain and Body— the Endocannabinoid System

Research on cannabis' effects led to the discovery of a biochemical communication system in the human body called the endocannabinoid system (ECS). This system has been found to play a crucial role in regulating our physiology, mood, and everyday experience. For example, the euphoric sensation called "runner's high" is induced through the ECS.

Specific receptors in the brain have been found to respond to cannabinoids – chemical compounds that trigger cannabinoid receptors. The identification of endogenous cannabinoid compounds has significantly advanced our understanding of human biology, health, and disease. One example is arachidonoylethanolamine (AEA), a fatty acid neurotransmitter produced by our own bodies. Another name for AEA is anandamide, named after the Sanskrit word for bliss.

While endocannabinoids are found in the body, exogenous cannabinoids are compounds which originated outside the body- for example, those from the cannabis plant. They can modulate many physiological systems in the human brain and body, including the neurological, immune, and hormonal systems. Evidence shows that cannabinoids can reduce inflammation, modify pain perception, increase appetite, and prolong deep sleep.

Benefits, Methods, and Status of CBD Use

Cannabinoids are a group of varied but related compounds found in cannabis. There are at least 120 different cannabinoids that have been isolated from the cannabis plant. The best studied cannabinoids include tetrahydrocannabinol (THC), cannabidiol (CBD), and cannabinol (CBN). Of all the cannabinoids, CBD is by far the most researched and marketed product. It acts as a neuromodulator for a variety of processes, including motor learning, appetite, and pain sensation, among other cognitive and physical processes.

The most commonly used form of CBD is CBD oil. By combining CBD extract with a carrier oil like coconut oil it can be ingested, vaped, or applied as a topical. Most CBD products contain less than 0.4% THC and thus are considered a food product. However, federally the U.S. Drug Enforcement Administration (DEA) continues to classify CBD as a Schedule I drug. Therefore, it's illegal unless you live in a state that has legalized medical and recreational use of marijuana. Check with your state law to be sure you are complying with the law. Many states require patients to obtain a prescription from a medical doctor to purchase and use cannabis products.

CBD Found to be Effective, and Safe from Dependency or Abuse

CBD is a non-psychoactive cannabis component that reduces pain, inflammation, and anxiety. It is free of the compound that causes one to get high from THC, while boosting cannabis' other beneficial effects. The effectiveness of CBD in human clinical trials has been demonstrated to help reduce:

- Chronic neuropathic pain
- Spasticity
- Insomnia
- Bladder problems (from multiple sclerosis)
- Nausea
- Cancer related pain
- Rheumatoid arthritis symptoms

Studies also showed that no tolerance to CBD developed, no dose escalation was necessary, and no evidence of drug dependence or withdrawal was seen in patients taking the medicine for one to four years. After initial dosage adjustment, patients achieved effective symptom control without notable psychoactive effects. Patients were able to carry on with daily living, and it sometimes allowed a previously-debilitated patient to return to work or school. No reports of abuse or diversion of CBD have occurred in clinical trials, long term extension studies, or general prescription use.

Cannabis Is Effective for Chemo-Induced Nausea and Vomiting

Since 1985, synthetic cannabinoids marketed under the names dronabinol and nabilone have been approved by the FDA for treatment of Chemotherapy Induced Nausea and Vomiting (CINV). Subsequently, nearly 30 clinical trials have been conducted and show that synthetic cannabinoids are superior to traditional dopamine antagonists, drugs which block dopamine receptors in the brainstem and therefore reduce symptoms of nausea and vomiting. Common dopamine antagonist drugs include Raglan, Compazine, and Thorazine.

In recent years, preliminary studies and anecdotal reports have shown that naturally derived CBD may achieve the same effectiveness as synthetic cannabinoids but with fewer side effects. It helps relieve CINV but without such side effects as:

- Drowsiness
- Depression
- Drops in blood pressure
- Hallucinations
- Paranoia

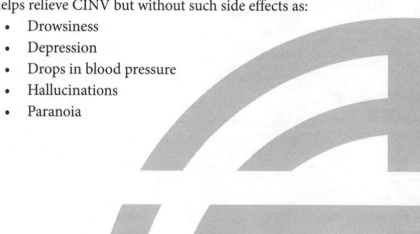

An FDA Approved CBD Product for Seizure Disorders

In the past, the FDA has approved several drugs for appetite stimulation and pain regulation. They were synthesized cannabinoids with names like Marinol, Syndros, and Nabilone. Very recently, the FDA approved Epidiolex. Epidiolex is CBD naturally derived from the cannabis plant to treat two rare and severe forms of epilepsy. This marked the first time a non-synthetic cannabinoid had been approved in the United States.

However, the first regulatory approval for a naturally-derived cannabis product in North America was given by Health Canada for Nabiximols (Sativex). It is used for symptomatic relief of neuropathic pain and muscle spasticity from multiple sclerosis. Nabiximols is a formulated extract of cannabis sativa with a THC:CBD ratio of 1:1.

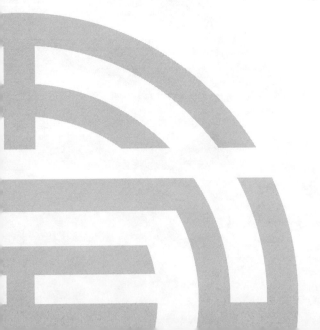

Cannabinoids Found Effective for Neuropathy

Neuropathic pain, or neuropathy, is a worldwide epidemic that occurs in 3% to 8% of individuals in industrialized countries. Existing treatments have been inadequate, often interfering with sleep and affecting overall quality of life. Neuropathy disproportionately affects cancer patients who have undergone chemotherapy and suffered corresponding chemo-induced nerve damage in their extremities. The drugs currently available to treat neuropathic pain are, at best, moderately effective, and some have intolerable side effects. Recent research of cannabinoids shows promising results for neuropathy.

Data from large, well-controlled studies over the last five years shows that cannabinoids are moderately effective in reducing chronic pain. This suggests that cannabinoids can play a useful role in the management of chronic nerve pain.

CB1 and CB2 Are Receptors and Not Radios

There are receptors throughout the human brain and body that interact with cannabinoids. The two primary ones are:

- CB1 - found mostly in neurons in the brain and central nervous system.
- CB2 - found mainly in the immune system and related organs such as the spleen, tonsils, and thymus gland. These receptors work like a lock and key when flooded with cannabinoids.

Since CB1 receptors are mostly located in the brain and central nervous system, they are particularly sensitive to THC. THC has been shown to possess a very high binding affinity with CB1 receptors. Therefore, high THC products provide quick relief from pain, nausea, or depression, especially for cancer patients undergoing chemotherapy.

CB2 receptors on the other hand are located in the immune system, including the gastrointestinal lining where they modulate intestinal inflammatory response. This may be why sufferers of Crohn's disease and IBS respond so well to CBD products. The benefits also extend to patients suffering from inflammation like arthritis and lupus.

Each Person's Differing Cannabinoid Sensitivity

Researchers have observed how different patients with specific diseases have different expressions of CB1 and CB2 receptors than patients who are not afflicted with these conditions. The variations in cannabinoid receptors in an individual results in a range of responses to different cannabis products.

When a patient over expresses a receptor and overacts to a cannabinoid, such as THC, the formulator must carefully dose by starting with a smaller concentration. When another patient under expresses a receptor, they may need to consume greater quantities or add other cannabinoids and terpenes to the mix to achieve the desired relief. This is the reason that it's essential for patients to seek out only experienced and expert formulators. It is a formulator's job to find just the right combination tailored to your cannabinoid receptor expression and your health needs.

CBD Found Effective for Generalized Anxiety Disorder

In recent years, CBD has drawn increasing interest as a treatment for a range of neuropsychiatric disorders. Several studies provide strong evidence that supports CBD as a treatment for:

- Generalized anxiety disorder
- Panic disorder
- Social anxiety disorder
- Obsessive–compulsive disorder
- Post-traumatic stress disorder

However, few studies have focused on CBD for chronic anxiety disorder and its appropriate long term dosing. Overall, current evidence indicates CBD has considerable potential as a treatment for multiple anxiety disorders.

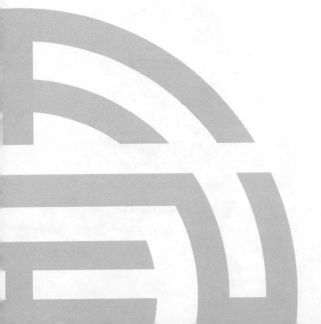

More Ways to Consume CBD Products

After consulting with your doctor and formulator about trying CBD, you'll need to decide on a consumption method. The main consideration will be the onset time, the relief duration, and whether you are looking for systemic or localized relief. Systemic relief affects the whole body, whereas localized relief only affects the area which the product was applied, such as a CBD rub. Often, a combined systemic and localized approach is the best way.

For example, you can use a CBD infused rub to relieve arthritic pain in your joints along with a systemic CBD tincture to reduce inflammation, which is the root of the condition. The complementary approach takes into account that some products provide instant relief for a short amount of time, while others have a longer onset time but provide relief for a longer period of time. Again, it's important to work with an experienced, licensed healthcare professional who can help tailor the right product combination at the right dosage for you. This way you receive the maximum benefit and minimum undesirable effects.

Localized CBD Delivery Systems

This category of products is often referred to as topicals. Some only impact the skin layer to which they are applied, while others penetrate into the muscles and joints underneath the skin. Localized delivery systems of cannabinoids include rubs, roll-on oils, sprays, and bath soaks.

Rubs and roll-ons contain CBD infusions that are applied directly to the skin for localized relief of pain and inflammation. They are perfect for treating muscle, joint, and surface level pain, and relief is often felt in as little as 15 minutes. Sprays are another form of CBD infused topical that are sprayed directly onto the skin for those suffering from painful skin conditions like shingles, eczema, or psoriasis. Some sprays even act as beauty products to help reduce wrinkles and rejuvenate the skin. Bath soaks are CBD infused bath salts that induce a calming and soothing effect. Often times they are combined with essential oils to enhance the therapeutic intent. Besides its relaxation property, bath soaks can also be used for generalized body tension, tightness, and pain.

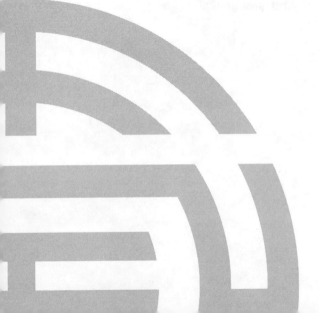

Systemic CBD Delivery Systems

For consistent relief of pain, inflammation, anxiety, and appetite stimulation, patients often benefit from ingesting a daily dose of CBD. Oral administration of cannabis products come in a dizzying array of forms, including tinctures, capsules, powders, edibles, and smokeables.

A tincture is a liquid CBD extract either in an alcohol or oil base that is applied under the tongue. The extract is absorbed by the artery under the tongue within seconds and bypasses the digestive tract. However, the full extent of the effects can take up to an hour to be felt.

Capsules contain a CBD extract either in powder form or in an organic oil, such as MCT coconut oil carrier. These capsules have a longer onset time as they need to pass through the digestive tract to be absorbed. Powders or isolates are pure CBD crystals that are easily vaporized.

Edibles are CBD infused candies, cookies, brownies, and much more. The effects are similar to capsules since the extract must be absorbed by the digestive tract.

Finally, smokeables are the good, old-fashioned marijuana joint or bong hit. We highly discourage smokeables due to the difficulty of ensuring a consistent dose of CBD, THC, and terpenes, as well as the negative impact it has on the respiratory system.

Tinctures, capsules, and edibles provide the longest relief. They can last anywhere between 4 to 8 hours, depending on the individual's cannabinoid receptor expression. On the other hand, vaporizing CBD isolate provides the fastest systemic relief, lasting from 2 to 4 hours depending on the individual. Again, always work with an expert on determining the best form for your specific condition.

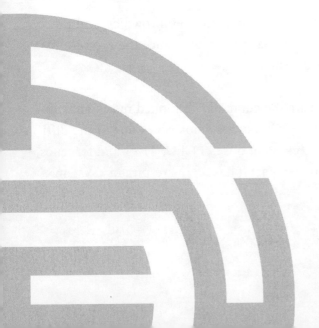

You've Had Plenty of Whiffs of Terpenoids

As an aromatic compound in plants, many terpenoids or terpenes are familiar to our noses. For example:
- Pinene emits the scent of pine trees or turpentine.
- Linalool is commonly found in lavender, whose essential oil is commonly used to soothe anxiety and depression.
- Limonene, found in the rinds of citrus, assists the healing of skin and mucous membranes.

These and many other terpenes found in cannabis have profound therapeutic benefits. Terpinolene is found to possess antioxidant and anticancer properties, valencene has anti-inflammatory actions, and bisabolol has been shown in recent research to induce apoptosis or programmed cell death in leukemia cells. This is just to name a few.

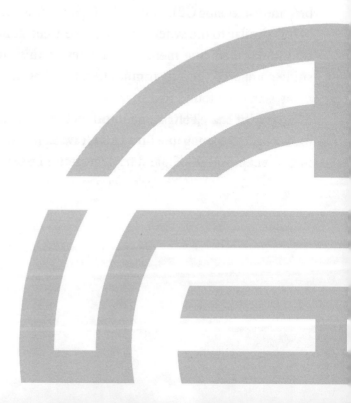

The Entourage Effect of Terpenes

Amongst the hundreds of organic compounds found in cannabis, one of the most important is the terpenes. Terpenes are the volatile oils that provide the plant with strong aromas and color that are meant to deter insects and herbivores. In cannabis, terpenes provide cannabis its unique aroma, like the notes in fine wine. Terpenes are the major component in most essential oils. The contents of the volatile oil depend on the genotype, sunlight, environmental conditions, developmental stage, and breeding methods used on the plant.

Why are terpenes important? Studies show that when different terpenes are combined with different cannabinoids, the result is the entourage effect. The entourage effect means that synergistic use of cannabinoids and terpenes produce greater therapeutic benefits than using CBD and/or THC alone. Another way to think of it is similar to the synergistic effect between conventional and traditional medicine mentioned earlier in this book. A recent study compared the anti-tumor effects of THC alone to a whole plant extract. It found that the whole plant cannabis extract was more potent than THC alone in cell culture and animal models of Estrogen Receptor positive (ER+), human epidermal growth factor receptor (HER+), and triple negative breast cancer.

Enhanced Terpenes Achieve
Better Symptom Relief with Chinese Herbs

Since ancient China, physicians have understood the synergistic power that arises when two or more combined ingredients yield an amplified benefit. This is the case for CBD infused with Chinese herbal medicine to help manage the symptoms of cancer, both during treatment and afterwards. Five symptoms managed very well with CBD herbal infusion include:

- Stomach distress
- Pain
- Insomnia
- Anxiety
- Fatigue

Below are the herbs that are most effective for each symptom.

- For nausea include ginger, Chinese basil, and cardamom.
- For pain include corydalis, myrrh, and frankincense.
- For insomnia include jujube seed, biota, and polygala.
- For anxiety and depression include mimosa bark, bupleurum, and ginkgo.
- For fatigue and cognitive decline include astragalus, goji berry, and cordyceps.

Most Chinese herbs contain very high levels of terpenoids, which is advantageous when it comes to CBD enhanced actions.

A special process is required to infuse Chinese herbal extracts into CBD tinctures in order to achieve quality and efficacy. First the herbal formula must be extracted on low heat with MCT coconut oil, which is a carrier oil for CBD extract. Then the two extracts must be blended carefully and expertly in an ideal temperature in order to produce the ultimate synergy.

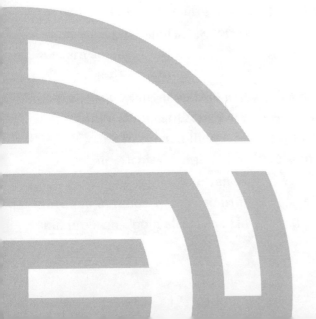

To Sativa or Indica—That Is the Question

The cannabis plant has two main species: cannabis sativa and cannabis indica. They contain more than 400 identified chemicals, including cannabidiol (CBD), tetrahydrocannabinol (THC), terpenoids, and flavonoids. Each species has its own range of effects on the body and mind, resulting in a wide range of medicinal benefits. Some botanists have claimed that indica strains generally provide a sense of deep body relaxation, while sativa strains tend to provide a more energizing experience. The sedative effects of indica strains is falsely attributed to CBD content when, in fact, CBD is stimulating in low and moderate doses!

Different effects are observed amongst different cannabis species due to their terpenoid content. The sedation property in most cannabis is attributable to their myrcene content, a terpene with a strongly sedative effect that resembles a narcotic. In contrast, a high limonene content will be uplifting to mood. The presence of the relatively rare terpene alpha-pinene can effectively reduce or eliminate the short-term memory impairment classically induced by THC. In summary, it's important to know not only the CBD and THC content of a product you are considering taking, but also the types and amounts of terpenoids present. This will help to enhance the positive benefits.

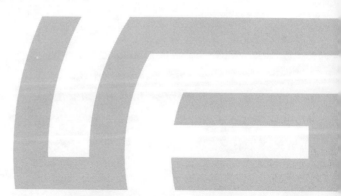

Rick Simpson, CBD Oil, and Basal Cell Carcinoma

A well-known, anecdotal case posted on the internet involved the use of cannabis products for treating cancer. Rick Simpson chose to treat his basal cell carcinoma (skin cancer) lesions topically with a concentrated cannabis oil. After repeated applications, it was reported the cancer lesions disappeared.

Since it is an anecdotal report instead of the gold standard of a double-blind study, the medical community gives no credence to the report. However, Rick Simpson's case report does warrant further research. This is especially true after cell line and animal model research suggests that CB1 and CB2 receptors, which cannabinoids specifically bind to, can inhibit angiogenesis (new blood vessel growth) in skin cancers. Studies are ongoing.

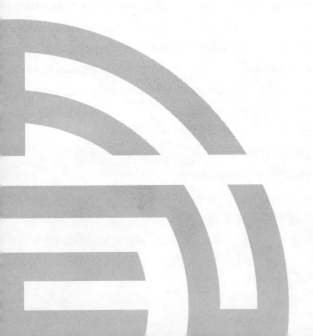

CBD Increased Survival Time for Those with Glioblastoma

Two prospective clinical trials have been conducted involving CBD and THC in an attempt to examine their anti-cancer properties and safety for patients with glioblastoma multiforme, an aggressive brain cancer. The control group took chemotherapy and placebos, while the study group was given the same chemotherapy along with a 1:1 THC:CBD product. When compared, the study group had a higher 1-year survival rate than the control group.

Antiproliferative effects were recorded in some of the patients. The combination of THC and CBD with the chemo drug temozolomide appears to be safe, but a larger phase II study is recommended.

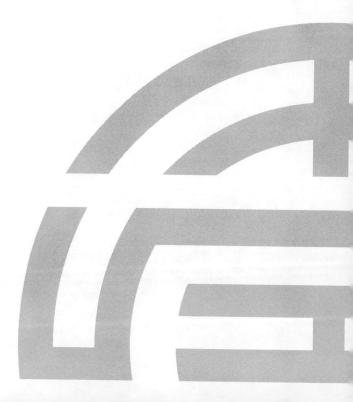

Cannabis Found Generally Synergistic with Chemotherapy

A number of preclinical studies have tested whether there would be conflict or synergy combining cannabis with chemotherapy drugs. In studies on lung, colon, pancreatic, brain, and gastric cancer cell cultures, using chemo drugs like paclitaxel or gemcitabine had no observable adverse herb-drug interactions and synergy was common. Likewise, cannabis extract was found to be synergistic with tamoxifen, lapatinib, and cisplatin chemotherapy in breast cancer cells and animal tests.

These and other studies provide reassuring data for cancer patients who wish to integrate cannabis into their conventional treatment to reduce side effects.

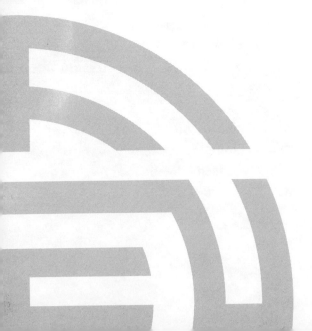

Three Main Types of Cannabis Products

In general, there are three types of cannabis products depending on their concentrations of THC and CBD:

- Type 1 is THC-dominant, it contains high levels of THC and low concentrations of CBD, this causes strong psychoactive effects.
- Type 2 is a mixed combination of varying parts of THC and CBD, it produces some psychoactive changes with the benefits of CBD.
- Type 3 is CBD-dominant, it has high concentrations of CBD and low THC content, which means no euphoric effects.

According to Israeli research, the therapeutic synergy seen in plant extracts means less active components are needed, resulting in reduced adverse side effects. In other words, full spectrum CBD cannabis oil is effective at much lower doses and has a wider therapeutic window than a CBD-isolate or a primarily THC cannabis product.

Understanding Dosing for Mixed THC and CBD Products

Once you understand CB1 (brain and nervous system) and CB2 (immune and gut) receptors and the binding strength of THC and CBD on each receptor, it's easy to figure out the combination ratio of the two for a patient's unique needs.

More THC means:
- Higher psychoactivity
- Increased appetite
- Relieved stress and anxiety
- Reduced inflammation
- Relaxation and euphoria

The more CBD, the better for:
- Autoimmune disorders
- Arthritis
- Psoriasis
- Gastrointestinal issues (such as Crohn's and colitis)

For instance, a 1:3 ratio of CBD:THC will most likely produce a calming sensation with reduced anxiety and stress, while promoting anti-inflammatory and pain relief. A ratio of 1:1 CBD:THC shows promise in relieving symptoms associated with multiple sclerosis and may also be able to inhibit certain cancer cells and tumor growth. CBD dominant ratios of 20:1 or 1:0 result in no psychoactivity and may be most effective for curbing seizures, anxiety, psychosis, PTSD, and neurodegenerative conditions such as Parkinson's and Huntington's Disease.

Again, we strongly advise anyone who is considering adding cannabis to their health regimen to consult with their primary care physician or specialist before taking medical marijuana.

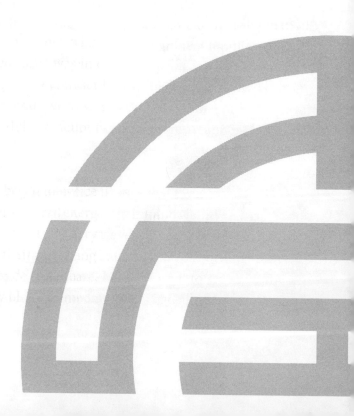

General Dosing Guidelines for THC

Average-sized adult patients with little or no prior experience using cannabis are advised to start slowly, with 1 to 2 mg of THC shortly before bedtime for two days. If there are no unwanted side effects, increase the bedtime dose of THC by another 1 to 2 mg for the next two days. Continue to increase the dose of THC by an additional 1 to 2 mg every other day until the desired calming and sedative effects are achieved. If there are adverse side effects, reduce the dose of THC to the prior, well tolerated amount.

According to a report published in Nature, oral administration of a low dose of THC (1 mg/day) resulted in "significant inhibition of disease progression" in an animal test of atherosclerosis (hardening of the arteries). This dose is lower than the dose usually associated with psychotropic effects of THC. Doses exceeding 20-30 mg of THC per day may increase adverse effects or build a tolerance without helping.

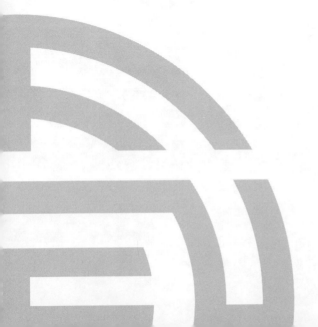

Lower Dose Cannabis Works Better Than Higher Dose for Cancer Pain

A clinical study published in the Journal of Pain examined the efficacy of different dosage levels of Sativex, a cannabis-derived sublingual spray with 1:1 CBD:THC ratio. It is an approved medication in two dozen countries, but not in the United States. The study followed 263 cancer patients who were not finding pain relief with opiates. The group that received 21 mg of Sativex each day experienced significant improvements in pain levels, more so than the group that received 52 mg Sativex daily.

Participants who were given even higher doses at 83 mg daily found their pain reduced even less than by placebo, and they experienced more adverse effects. The results show that often less is more when it comes to cannabis dosing. However, since each person is different, our advice is to work with a knowledgeable and licensed healthcare provider to find just the right dose and combination of cannabinoids for your condition.

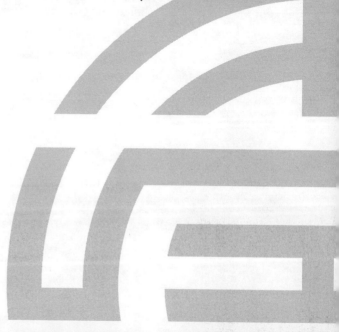

General Dosing Considerations for Cannabis

Each person is endowed with different CB1 and CB2 receptor expression; in other words everyone has different levels of sensitivity to cannabinoids. Because of this, it is important to consider the following when starting out – hopefully under the direct supervision and advice of a knowledgeable, licensed healthcare provider.

The three considerations are:
1. Is the patient a new or chronic user? Chronic users may need to take a break to resensitize their receptors.
2. Different ratios of CBD:THC should be employed depending on the time of day; higher CBD during the day and higher THC at night. For example, a daytime ratio may be 10:1, whereas at night it may change to 2:1.
3. Preventive low dosing can be employed to manage chronic symptoms like pain or limit further damage, such as for traumatic brain injury or heart attack.

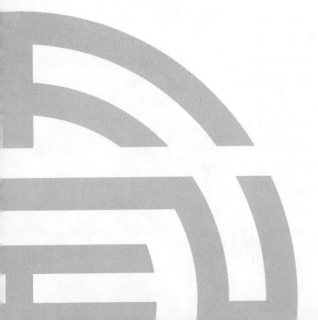

Speak to Your Doctor About Whether Cannabis Is Right for You

You may have heard about all the virtues and benefits of cannabis products and wondered whether it may also be good for your condition. Perhaps you're looking to reduce medications that are causing you unpleasant side effects. It's important to discuss with your doctor the use of any herbs or supplements, especially cannabis products, so that you can work together to achieve your health goals.

Before you go into the appointment, it's important to be clear about what you want to discuss with your doctor. Why do you want to take CBD? Are you experiencing problems or side effects with your current medication that you'd like to get off of? What symptoms are you looking to get relief for? Anxiety? Pain? Insomnia? Do you have any concerns about using CBD products? Keep in mind that the medical establishment tends to lag behind the latest developments and advances, so be patient and bring evidence-based literature to help educate and bring your doctor up to date.

Watch out for Cannabis-Drug Interactions

Despite it being one of the safest substances, CBD inhibits the activity of an enzyme called cytochrome P450. P450 is responsible for metabolizing many of the compounds you put into your body, including about 60% of the drugs you consume. When CBD slows down the activity of this enzyme, it takes longer to do its job. This can raise the level of a drug in your system, as well as extending the length of time it takes your body to process it.

Drugs that can be affected by CBD include:
- Anesthetics
- Blood pressure lowering medications
- Beta-blockers
- Analgesics
- Antibiotics
- Anti-seizure medications
- As well as other medications.

Always check with your doctor or pharmacist before combining cannabis products with any drugs you have been prescribed.

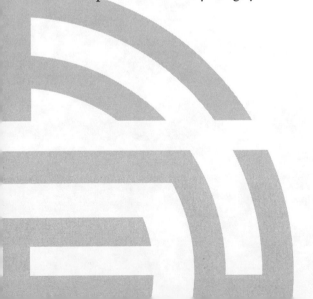

Resources and Products

DISCLAIMER:
THE AUTHORS COMPILED THIS SECTION FEATURING PRODUCTS AND INFORMATION RESOURCES BASED ON THEIR RESEARCH AND EXPERIENCE FOR THE CONVENIENCE OF THE READER. THE INFORMATION CONTAINED WITHIN IS FOR EDUCATIONAL PURPOSES AND DOES NOT CONSTITUTE MEDICAL ADVICE. READERS ARE ADVISED TO CHECK WITH THEIR DOCTORS BEFORE BEGINNING ANY PRODUCTS AND PROGRAMS MENTIONED HEREIN AND THROUGHOUT THE BOOK. THE STATEMENTS DESCRIBING THE PRODUCTS IN THIS SECTION HAVE NOT BEEN EVALU-ATED BY THE FDA. THESE PRODUCTS ARE NOT INTENDED TO DIAGNOSE, TREAT, CURE OR PREVENT DISEASE.

Dealing with cancer is more than a full time job! This is why we have compiled a list of resources all in one place, ranging from diet and nutrition with easy to prepare recipes to fresh and organically prepared food delivery services. Other helpful resources include herbal and nutraceutical formulas and ingredients, aromatherapy, qi gong and meditation that are mentioned in the book.

Additionally, we have listed selected online websites for more information on acupuncture and Chinese medicine, integrative approaches to cancer care as well as latest research on cutting edge diagnostic and treatment techniques for cancer. We have also included Tao of Wellness' telemedicine consultation services to help patients, especially those who can't visit one of our offices.

Consultations integrate oncology plans in collaboration with their oncologists, diet and nutrition plans, as well as personalized formulations for herbal and CBD protocols.

Finally, prevention of cancer or its recurrence is ultimately what we want for ourselves and our family, therefore we have also included books and distance-learning courses on nutrition, health, self improvement and feng shui, as well as an accredited school of Chinese medicine cofounded by Dr. Mao for those inspired to serve others by pursuing a career as a doctor of acupuncture and Chinese medicine.

Information Sites

LiveLongLiveStrongNow.com
The official website for this book with regular updates on research, studies and resources related to aging and cancer, Chinese medicine and other complementary modalities that comprise the practice of integrative oncology. You will also find various dietary menu plans specific for cancer prevention as well as for while going through cancer treatments.

Cancer Support Community (cancersupportcommunity.org)
As the largest professionally led nonprofit network of cancer support worldwide, the Cancer Support Community (CSC) is dedicated to ensuring that all people impacted by cancer are empowered by knowledge, strengthened by action, and sustained by community. This global network of 175 locations, including CSC and Gilda's Club centers, health-care partnerships, and satellite locations that deliver more than $50 million in free support services to patients and families.

National Cancer Institute (cancer.gov)

The National Cancer Institute (NCI) is part of the National Institutes of Health (NIH), which is one of eleven agencies that are part of the U.S. Department of Health and Human Services. The NCI coordinates the United States National Cancer Program and conducts and supports research, training, health information dissemination, and other activities related to the causes, prevention, diagnosis, and treatment of cancer; the supportive care of cancer patients and their families; and cancer survivorship.

Memorial Sloan Kettering Cancer Center (mskcc.org)

Memorial Sloan Kettering Cancer Center (MSK or MSKCC) is a cancer treatment and research institution in New York City, founded in 1884 as the New York Cancer Hospital. MSKCC is the largest and oldest private cancer center in the world, and is one of 47 National Cancer Institute-designated Comprehensive Cancer Centers. It offers integrative oncology treatment modalities onsite.

MD Anderson Cancer Center (mdanderson.org)

The University of Texas MD Anderson Cancer Center (colloquially MD Anderson) is one of the original three comprehensive cancer centers in the United States. It is both a degree-granting academic institution, and a cancer treatment and research center located at the Texas Medical Center in Houston. It is affiliated with The University of Texas Health Science Center at Houston.

Dana-Farber Cancer Institute (dana-farber.org)

Dana–Farber Cancer Institute is a comprehensive cancer treatment and research center in Boston, Massachusetts. It is a principal teaching affiliate of Harvard Medical School, and a founding member of the Dana–Farber/ Harvard Cancer Center, a Comprehensive Cancer Center designated by the National

Cancer Institute.

Moffitt Cancer Center (moffitt.org)

H. Lee Moffitt Cancer Center & Research Institute is a nonprofit cancer treatment and research center located in Tampa, Florida. Established in 1981 by the Florida Legislature, the hospital opened in October 1986, on the University of South Florida campus. Moffitt is the only National Cancer Institute-designated Comprehensive Cancer Center based in Florida.

Mayo Clinic Cancer Center (mayoclinic.org/departments-centers/mayo-clinic-cancer-center)

The Mayo Clinic Cancer Center is an NCI-designated Cancer Center and a division of the Mayo Clinic. The MCCC has 3 locations in the United States: Phoenix, Arizona, Jacksonville, Florida, and Rochester, Minnesota. The Mayo Clinic Cancer Center is one of the oldest NCI-designated cancer centers in the US, having first been designated in 1973.

City of Hope Cancer Center (cityofhope.org)

City of Hope is a private, not-for-profit clinical research center, hospital and graduate medical school located in Duarte, California, United States. The center's main campus resides on 110 acre of land adjacent to the boundaries of Duarte and Irwindale, with a network of clinical practice locations throughout Southern California, satellite offices in Monrovia and Irwin- dale, and regional fundraising offices throughout the United States. City of Hope is best known as a cancer treatment center. It has been designated a Comprehensive Cancer Center by the National Cancer Institute.

The Angeles Clinic (theangelesclinic.org)

The Angeles Clinic & Research Institute in West Los Angeles,

California has a staff of board-certified medical oncologists, radiologists, surgeons, immunotherapists, pathologists, and dermatologists. The cancer specialists at the Angeles Clinic use PET/CT, radiofrequency ablation, radiology oncology imaging services, clinical trials to provide advanced care for cancer of the brain, ovary, bladder, uterine, breast, cervix, GI, head & neck, lung, skin, prostate, bladder, and testicle. The center's hematologists and oncologists also specialize in treating anemia, leukemia, melanoma, lymphoma and plasma cell disorders.

American Cancer Society (cancer.org)

The American Cancer Society (ACS) is a nationwide voluntary health organization dedicated to eliminating cancer. Established in 1913, the society is organized into eleven geographical divisions of both medical and lay volunteers operating in more than 900 offices throughout the United States. Its home office is located in the American Cancer Society Center in Atlanta, Georgia. The ACS publishes the journals Cancer, CA: A Cancer Journal for Clinicians and Cancer.

Pink Lotus Breast Center (pinklotus.com)

Founded by Dr. Kristi Funk, The Pink Lotus Breast Center is a comprehensive and integrative breast center exclusively dedicated to the prevention, screening, diagnosis and treatment of breast cancer. Expedited scheduling; quick answers; less stress; top doctors; female-run; not hospital-owned; no facility fees; and a single location for all of your breast health needs.

Susan G. Komen foundation (komen.org)

From its inception in 1982 up to 2010, Komen has spent nearly $1.5 billion for breast cancer education, research, advocacy, health services and social support programs in the U.S., and through partnerships in more than 50 countries. Today, Komen has more than 100,000 volunteers working in a network of 124 affiliates worldwide. A non-profit organization focused on breast cancer that is devoted to advancing research and information sharing and community building for breast cancer patients, cancer survivors and their family. partnerships in more than 50 countries. Today, Komen has more than 100,000 volunteers working in a network of 124 affiliates worldwide. A non-profit organization focused on breast cancer that is devoted to advancing research and information sharing and community building for breast cancer patients, cancer survivors and and their family.

Nutritional and Chinese Herbal Supplements (WellnessLivingStore.com)

Wellness Living Store offers high quality health and wellness products ranging from herbal formulas passed down from Dr. Mao's family lineage, nutritional supplements to aromatherapy, books on health and spirituality, instructional audio and video programs on meditation, qi gong and tai chi. It also offers feng shui products to uplift your home and workplace energy.

Organic Prepared Food Delivery (EatNBeWell.com)

Delicious and organic prepared meals delivered to your door that feature specific menu plans for supporting cancer patients before, during and after their treatments as well as recipes featuring foods that research have shown to lower risks of cancer occurrence and recurrence.

Acupuncture & Chinese Medicine (acupuncture.com)

A comprehensive information site that provides everything you want to know about acupuncture and Chinese medicine ranging from diet and nutrition, acupuncture, tuina bodywork and acupressure, cupping, and Chinese herbal medicine. It provides content for both professionals and consumers alike as well as referrals for licensed acupuncture and Chinese medicine doctors.

Yo San University (YoSan.edu)

Yo San University is a nonprofit organization that educates students to become exceptional practitioners of Traditional Chinese Medicine and the Taoist healing arts. The school facilitates the development of students' spiritual and professional growth, and provides the community with an award-winning integrative medical care model and services. It offers rigorous, accredited Masters Degree program in acupuncture and Chinese medicine and Clinical Doctoral program in women's health, reproductive medicine and integrative medicine/healthy aging & longevity. Yo San University nurtures a lifelong career that expresses your compassion and desire to serve others.

Natural Pet Care Products (HerbalPetCare.org)

Herbal Pet Care is a collaborative project between Yo San University of Traditional Chinese Medicine and Voice for the Animals, both nonprofit organizations. It was conceived to bring natural care and restore vitality to pets which are part of our human family. The herbal formulations include non-toxic, natural herbs for fleas, skin problems, digestive conditions, immune and cancer support, and arthritis to name a few. They come from thousands of years of experience in caring for animals in the Chinese medicine tradition. Net proceeds go to support the wonderful work of these two organizations.

Diet, Nutrition & Herbal Supplements
(Available online at WellnesLivingStore.com)

Prepared Food delivery Service (getwelleating.com)

It's not easy cooking for yourself, let alone cooking for your entire family when you are busy with work and life and recovering from illness. Now there's an easier way—a fully prepared, ready to eat organic meals of pre-planned menu curated by Dr. Mao or your choices, delivered to your doors at an affordable price for you and your entire family. It's also a wonderful way to show your love by gifting it to someone you care that's going through cancer treatments. Use code LIVELONG for a 20% discount on first order.

Thymus Support

The major function of thymus is to produce natural killer cells (NK) that target virus, bacteria, fungus and cancer cells. With the aging process the thymus atrophies and therefore its critical immune support function declines. The unique nutrients in Thymus Support promote resistance to disease and cancer, guard against infections by stimulating white blood cells, and are effective in detoxifying microbial toxins and heaven metal poisoning. Thymus Support contains: colostrum, bee pollen, astragalus, and glandular extracts of thymus, spleen, lymph, bone marrow and adrenal gland sourced from New Zealand's grass grazing, organic cows.

YSJG granules

The Chinese herbal formula being used in the Beijing Cancer Hospital for breast cancer patients suffering from muscle and joint pain due to aromatase inhibitor drugs. Its efficacy has been confirmed in a study published in the journal, Breast. It contains: rehmannia, cuscuta, cypress, ligustici, corydalis, trachelospermum, and other herbs. Patients treated with YSJG granules showed significant pain reduction after 12 and 24 weeks. Improvements in physical, social/family, emotional, and functional well-being were seen as well. Moreover, YSJG granules did not increase serum estradiol levels.

Mushroom 10X
The most potent medicinal mushroom formula available. Combining lions mane, chaga, turkey tail, reishi, shiitake, agaricus, polyporus, poria, cordycep, and puffball in a synergistic blend that attains the maximum benefits of immune boosting powers of medicinal mushrooms.

Vitality
A clinical formula of vitality boosting herbs, such as astragalus, schisandra berry and goji berry to increase energy and stamina, especially helpful for patients undergoing cancer treatments dealing with side effects of fatigue and weakness.

Immunity
A formulation of natural Chinese herbs for a broad-spectrum balance to help nourish the body's natural immunity and to have soothing effects for a potent boost to maintain your vitality and health. Use at the first signs of lagging energy or use daily for immune support. Contains the following herbs: Japanese Honeysuckle, Forsythia, Kudzu, Apricot Kernel, White Mulberry, Burdock, Isatis, Schizonepeta, Siler, Soy Bean Seed, Notopterygium, Fragrant Angelica, Chinese Mint, Scrophularia, Licorice.

Probiotics
Not all probiotics are made equal. Most products on store shelves are DOA (dead on arrival). That's why we promote eating probiotic rich foods, such as cultured vegetables, like kimchi and sauerkraut, cultured plant milk, like coconut and almond kefir, and

fermented products, like miso, tempeh, and low sugar kombucha. However, if you like to supplement in addition to what you get in your diet, we recommend Wellness Living Probiotics for its high bioavailable and bioactive organisms. It contains: lactobacillus acidophilus, lactobacillus bifidus in a milk-free prebiotic base.

Inflammation Fighter
Cellular and tissue inflammation are at the root of many disease process ranging from arthritis, heart disease, diabetes, to cancer and obesity. It's like a wild fire in the body that when spreading out of control it can cripple essential functions leading to pain, mutations and organ failure. Inflammation Fighter taps nature's anti-inflammatory enzymes from papaya and pineapple to extinguish the inflammatory wild fire, reducing and preventing undesirable cellular and tissue damage. It contains: Papain, Bromelain as well as digestion-promoting betaine HCL, Pancreatin and glutamine. It can also be used as an excellent digestive aid.

Sugar Leveler
High blood glucose is implicated as a danger for nerve damage to the eye and extremities as well as to organs such as kidneys. In addition, it can result in elevated IGF-1, growth factor that may speed the development of cancer cells. Sugar Leveler was formulated to aid the body to control glucose metabolism and maintain normal blood sugar levels. It contains many crucial vitamins and minerals such as thiamine and chromium as well as alpha lipoid acid, aspartic acid, cinnamon, green tea, kelp and glandular extracts of pancreas, thyroid, liver, and adrenal gland sourced from New Zealand's grass grazing, organic cows.

Lymph Support
Keep your lymphatic system healthy to keep up the body's defense against infection and filter impurities from the body. Infection-

fighting white blood cells in the lymph nodes trap, attack and destroy foreign bacteria, virus, fungus and allergens. Give the body the nutrients it needs to keep the lymphatic system functioning well with Lymph Support. It contains: vitamin c, zinc, astragalus, burdock, goldenseal as well as glandular extracts of lymph and spleen sourced from New Zealand's grass grazing, organic cows.

Cell Protection

One of the major causes of aging and cancer is increased free radical damage—it has been likened to the process of rusting, breaking down function and leading to increased risk for disease and death. Cell Protection is a unique combination of potent antioxidants to help the body neutralize free radicals which comprise of viral and environmental toxins, pollutions, radiation and other damaging factors. Studies show that antioxidants can reduce the risk of many chronic diseases, such as cancer, cardiovascular disease, eye disease, Alzheimer's and Parkinson's Diseases. Cell Protection contains: lutein, lycopene, coenzyme Q10, grape seed extract, green tea extract, lipoid acid, superoxide dismutase and other antioxidants.

BSlim

Obesity has been implicated as a cause for increased cancer risks, especially that of the reproductive system. Specifically designed to easily integrate into your overall weight management program for effective results, the herbs in B-Slim were carefully selected by Dr. Mao according to the principles of Traditional Chinese Medicine and leave you with a healthy weight wellness aid. He has selected herbs whose qualities are said to control appetite and craving, eliminate bloating, improve digestion, increase fat metabolism, regulate blood sugar, gently relieve constipation and balance the body. Contains: Sacred Lotus Leaf, Green Tea

Leaf, Chinese Hawthorn Fruit, Chrysanthemum Flower, Chinese Salvia Root & Rhizome, White Mulberry Root Bark, Cang-zhu Atractylodes Rhizome, Radish Seed, Chinese Rhubarb Root & Rhizome, Pinella Rhizome, Fragrant Angelica Root.

Detox

Toxins are everywhere and studies have shown a direct link between certain environmental toxins such as bisphenol A in plastics, formaldehyde in adhesives and pesticides in food. Many of the toxins act as endocrine disruptors, increasing risks of reproductive cancers such as that of the breast, ovaries, uterus, and prostate. Chinese medicine has recognized the role environmental toxins played in health and disease, therefore protocols were developed to target the body's detoxification and elimination pathways mainly through the liver, kidneys and the skin. Detox was formulated to support the methylation and elimination of toxins through the urine, bowels and sweat. It contains oriental wormwood, golden grass, rhubarb, astragalus, daikon seed, plantain seed, Chinese basil, mint and other herbs.

CBD & Herbal Infusion (PureCBDHerb.com)

Combining the pure healing properties of CBD and Chinese herbs, Pure CBD Herb is a line of specially formulated blend of CBD tinctures infused with Chinese herbal extracts for various symptoms and health conditions. The line includes oral tinctures of CBD 300, CBD+Painless, CBD+Sleep, CBD+Calm, CBD+Immunity, CBD+Stomach, and topical CBD+Skin.

Qi Gong & Meditation Video/Audio (Downloadable on WellnessLivingStore.com)

Qi Gong Meditation for Cancer Support Video

This video learning program features Meditation and qi gong

specifically designed to aid your body's own ability to restore and maintain your health, while reducing side-effects caused by chemotherapy and radiation; these side effects can include fatigue, "brain fog," feeling down and anxious, digestive discomforts, and numbness or tingling in your hands and feet. These practices will empower you to activate your own healing powers, create a better quality of life and have a healthier outcome.

Calm Meditation Audio

In this audio learning program, you will learn the time-honored qi meditations and simple breathing exercises to significantly reduce anxiety and other personal issues in your body. You will tap into your body's own healing mechanisms to increase your immunity and prevent stress-related conditions.

Sleep Meditation Audio

This audio guided meditation program trains the mind to let go of words, thoughts, and images as you consciously welcome inner aware- ness and the stillness of deep sleep. This practice provides a guided meditation using simple breathing techniques and visualization to relax your body, while part one gives you vital information and tips to create a sleeping sanctuary and routine to train your body for restorative sleep.

Pain Release Meditation Audio

Learn mind-body techniques used by martial artists and Taoist monks intense training techniques that enabled them to endure and transcend excruciating pain. Throw pain away from your body as if throwing a ball. Abandon your limitations by outgrowing them. Overcome stiff- ness by mind-stretching your body as you've never been physically able to do. Use these simple visualization meditation exercises to aid you in the alleviation of pain. Draw on simple breathing and visualization techniques to keep yourself calm, peaceful and focused.

Feng Shui Five Elements Music Audio

Find balance in your life and invoke the power of the universe by using the Feng Shui Five Elements Musical Meditation. Designed to bring the transformative power of each element - Wood, Fire, Earth, Metal, and Water - to fill the missing Feng Shui spaces and welcome natural vibrations and energy into your home. This therapeutic music compilation is designed to counter elemental imbalances on physical, mindful and emotional levels. Each core Element track is a merging of sound vibration and healing that resonates with the organ system energies of that element. Ancient Chinese physicians were aware of the power of sound and music, therefore, they prescribed distinct harmonic therapies to help improve one's health. Revitalize your entire being by listening to the complete compilation. For Feng Shui application, adjust the energetic vibration of your living or working space by selecting tracks that correspond to the element space that you wish to nourish.

Six Healing Sounds Audio

This audio learning program guides you on a traditional Taoist meditation using sound and breathing exercises to clear your energetic meridians and reach a healthier state of mind and body. With this sound meditation you will learn the techniques to maintain a healthy state of mind that leads to a deeper sense of peace and happiness. In this program, Dr. Mao will guide you on understanding each sound that restores the energetic balance of the organ systems and with proper pronunciation of each healing sound so you too can harness this powerful aid for your own health and healing.

Taoist Meditation LIVE Online Course and Certification (CollegeOfTao.org)

Daily meditation is highly recommended by doctors for your health, by employers for your productivity, creativity, & ingenuity, and by spiritual teachers who know world peace begins with peace within yourself. Taoist meditation practices balance the body, mind, & spirit, deepening peace, personal power, and clarity.

Supported by thousands of years of case studies and several decades of modern scientific evidence, Taoist meditation practice offers an unparalleled experience of oneself as not only the drop of water in the ocean, but also the ocean in the drop of water. Taoist meditation philosophy is beautifully unique in its view of not only the human being in harmony, but the human being in harmony with all of existence.

Traditional Taoist meditation practice includes the universe, our environment, and our world in meditation, releasing the human being from ego isolation and welcoming our symbiotic, harmonious co-evolution with all of creation. The Taoist tradition emphasizes dialogue with a living teacher to be certain there is a complete understanding of practices and philosophy. Through questioning, inquiries, navigation of challenges, and application of meditation practice to daily life, a living teacher confirms your thorough understanding, emboldening your life and meditation practice.

For meditation to truly live on, this tradition of a human, living relationship between teacher and student must be kept alive. This online course is offered LIVE through Zoom conference and meets twice a month, an hour each time with daily practice expected by the students.

Books on Health, Healing and Longevity Available at (WellnessLivingStore.com)

Secrets of Longevity: Hundreds of Ways to Live to 100

Looking to live a longer, happier, healthier life? Try eating more blueberries, telling the truth, and saying no to undue burdens. These are just a few of the hundreds of tips profiled in Secrets of Longevity - a simple, no-nonsense approach to living longer. Dr. Mao Shing Ni, doctor to Hollywood stars and a Tai Chi master specializing in longevity, brings together simple and unusual ways to live longer in this beautifully designed, chunky paperback, putting at the fingertips a host of proven ways to make anyone's stay on earth much, much happier.

Secrets of Longevity Cook Book

There are over 80 delicious recipes which have "secret healing powers" selected from centenarians around the world. With a focus on using fresh foods that have specific health benefits and longevity properties, Dr. Mao highlights signature ingredients specific to each dish and provides an overview discussing the food's particular health benefits. Try these recipes and you will see a difference in your energy and heath! Also includes the following: Centenarians' Top Ten Habits for Good Health, List of Kitchen Essentials, Guide to Cookware for Longevity, Weekly Menus for Longevity and Health, and Spice & Herb Blends for 10 Common Health Conditions

Tao of Nutrition

The Tao of Nutrition provides information on making every meal therapeutic, teaching you how to make appropriate food choices for your ailments, your constitution, and the season of the year. This ancient knowledge from China provides guidance for the seasoned practitioner, as well as the new student of healthy living. By balancing your energies, the body heals itself. Balance is the key to health.

101 Vegetarian Delight

101 Vegetarian Delights is cooking based on the ancient Chinese tradition of balance and harmony. Recipes range from exotic flavorful feasts to nutritious everyday meals. Cooking with herbs, the culinary herb garden, and garnishing with beautiful edible flowers are also featured. Learn a natural way of eating that has both physical and spiritual benefits. Increase your joy of eating and move toward vibrant well-being as you expand your world of foods.

Chinese Vegetarian Delights

Being a vegetarian is the secret to longevity. This is because a plant-based diet has been proven to lower risks for heart disease, stroke and cancer—the top causes of death in modern times. Filled with delicious Asian-influenced recipes adapted for Western palate, Chinese Vegetarian Delights is a must for a vegetarian looking for delightful flavors that is at once tasty and therapeutic.

Secrets of Self Healing

Eastern medicine has long understood the extraordinary innate ability of the human body to fight disease and stay healthy. All it needs is an assist from natural measures-including time-tested disciplines like herbal therapy massage, and acupressure-to restore balance and stimulate healing from the inside out. In Secrets of Self-Healing, you'll discover self-care strategies at once steeped in Eastern wisdom and tradition and supported by modern science. Here's just a sampling: Allergies? Drink chamomile tea? Flu? Press a point near your thumb to stimulate defenses? Headache? Visualize relief with meditation technique? Insomnia? Soak feet before bedtime? Overweight?

Increase metabolism with apple cider vinegar? and much more!

Second Spring
The Chinese refer to a woman's midlife transition as her "Second Spring." Thanks to the simple, natural techniques of traditional Chinese medicine, the second half of a woman's life is a flowering of feminine potential rather than a physical and mental decline. Now, Dr. Mao's revolutionary Second Spring™ program gives you time-tested, completely natural treatments to enhance energy, sexuality, and health and initiate your own new season of vitality starting at age thirty-five, through pre-menopause, menopause, and beyond—all without the need for hormonal replacement therapy.

Power of Natural Healing
Heal yourself, or better yet, prevent problems in the first place. Revitalize health with acupuncture and herbs, Tai Chi, Chi Gong, sound, color, movement, visualization, breathing and meditation. A best seller at the Wellness Living Store.

Bibliography

Ch. 1: Why Does Cancer Happen?

Lawrence, M.S., Stojanov, P., Mermel, C.H., Robinson, J.T., Garraway, L.A., Golub, T.R., ...Getz, G. Discovery and saturation analysis of cancer genes across 21 tumour types. Nature. 2014. 505, 495-501.

Genetic Testing for Hereditary Cancer Syndromes. National Cancer Institute. Retrived from https://www.cancer.gov/about-cancer/causes-prevention/genetics/genetic-testing-fact-sheet#q2.

Volkan, O., Chung, W.K., The impact of hereditary cancer gene panels on clinical care and lessons learned. Cold Spring Harbor Molecular Case Studies. 2017. 3. (6): a002154

Soo You, J., & Jones, P.A., Cancer Genetics and Epigenetics: Two Sides of the Same Coin? Cancer Cell. 2012. 22 (1). 9-20.

Donaldson, M.S., Nutrition and cancer: A review of the evidence for an anti-cancer diet. Nutrition Journal. 2004.3, 19.

Bokyung, S., Sahdeo, P., Vivek, Y.R., Afsaneh, L., Bharat, A.B., Cancer and diet: How are they related? Free Radical Research. 45, 2011. 864-879.

Anand P, Kunnumakkara AB, Sundaram C, Harikumar KB, Tharakan ST, Lai OS, Sung B, Aggarwal BB. Cancer is a Preventable Disease that Requires Major Lifestyle Changes. Pharmaceutical Research. 2008. 25. (9). 2097–2116.

Diet, Nutrition, Physical Activity and Cancer: a Global Perspective. American Institute for Cancer Research. Retrieved from https://www.wcrf.org/dietandcancer.

Sieri, S., Agnoli, C., Pala, V., Grioni, S., Brighenti, F., Pellegrini, N., ... Krogh, V., Dietary glycemic index, glycemic load, and cancer risk: results from the EPIC-Italy study. Scientific Reports. 2017. 7. (1). 9757.

Sieri, S., Agnoli, C., Pala, V., Grioni, S., Brighenti, F., Pellegrini, N., ... Krogh, V., Dietary habits and cancer: the experience of EPIC-Italy. Epidemiologa e prevenzione. 2015. 39. (5-6). 333-8.

Cancer and diet: What's the connection? Harvard Health Publishing. Retrieved from https://www.health.harvard.edu/newsletters/harvard_mens_health_watch/2016/october

Lee, J.H., Khor, T.O., Shu, L., Su, Z.Y., Fuentes, F., Kong, A.N., Dietary phytochemicals and cancer prevention: Nrf2 signaling, epigenetics, and cell death mechanisms in blocking cancer initiation and progression. Pharmacology & Therapeutics. 2013. 137. (92). 153-171.

Vegetarian diet linked to lower colon cancer risk. Retrieved from, https://www.health.harvard.edu/blog/vegetarian-diet-linked-to-lower-colon-cancer-risk-201503117785

Patel, A., Pathak, Y., Patel, J., Sutariya, V., Role of nutritional factors in pathogenesis of cancer. Food Quality and Safety. 2018. 2. (1). 27-36.

Falasca, M., Casari, I., Maffucci, T., Cancer Chemoprevention With Nuts, JNCI: Journal of the National Cancer Institute. 2014. 106. (9).238.

Vogt, R., Bennett, D., Cassady, D., Frost, J., Ritz, B., Hertz-Picciotto, I. Cancer and non-cancer health effects from food contaminant exposures for children and adults in California: a risk assessment. Environmental Health. 2012. 11. 83.

Study finds high exposure to food-borne toxins. Preschool children are particularly vulnerable to compounds linked to cancer and other conditions. UC Davis Health. Retrieved from, https://health.ucdavis.edu/publish/news/cancer/7190

The Agency for Toxic Substances and Disease Registry (ATSDR). US Department of Health and Human Services.

Wogan GN, Hecht SS, Felton JS, Conney AH, Loeb LA. Environmental and chemical carcinogenesis. Seminar in Cancer Biology. 2004.14. (6). 473-86.

Field, R.W., DO, PhD, MS, & Withers, B.L., DO. Occupational and Environmental Causes of Lung Cancer. Clinics in Chest Medicine. 2012. 33. (4). 681-703.

Datzmann, T., Markevych, I., Trautmann, F., Heinrich J., Schmitt, J.., Tesch, F., Outdoor air pollution, green space, and cancer incidence in Saxony: a semi-individual cohort study. BMC Public Health. 2018. 18. (1). 715.

Brower, V., Tracking Chemotherapy's Effects on Secondary Cancers. JNCI: Journal of the National Cancer Institute. 2013. 105. (19). 1421-1422

Jones, M.E., van Leeuwen, F.E., Hoogendoorn, W.E., Mourits, M.JE., Hollema, H., van Boven, H.,... Swerdlow, A.J. Endometrial cancer survival after breast cancer in relation to tamoxifen treatment: Pooled results from three countries. Breast Cancer Research. 2012. 14. (3). R91.

Anand, P., Kunnumakara, A.B., Sundaram, C., Harikumar,K.B., Tharakan, S.T., Lai, O.S.,...Aggarwal, B.B. Cancer is a preventable disease that requires major lifestyle changes. Pharmaceutical Research. 2008. 25. (9). 2097-2116.

Tamoxifen and Raloxifene for Lowering Breast Cancer Risk. 2018. American Cancer Society. Retrieved from https://www.cancer.org/cancer/breast-cancer/risk-and-prevention/tamoxifen-and-raloxifene-for-breast-cancer-prevention.html

Channing J. Paller, C.J., & Thomas J. Smith, T.J. Finasteride and Prostate Cancer: A Commentary. Oncologist. 2012. 17. (7). 888-890.

Zhen Wang, Z., Chen, J., Jin-lu Liu, J., COX-2 Inhibitors and Gastric Cancer. Gastroenterology Research and Practice. 2014. Article ID 132320. 7 pages.

Mauney, M., (2018). Actos. Drugwatch. Retrieved from https://www.drugwatch.com/actos/

Zbuk, K., Anand, S.S., Declining incidence of breast cancer after decreased use of hormone-replacement therapy: magnitude and time lags in different countries. Journal of Epidemiology & Community Health. 2012. 66. (1). 1-7.

Ravdin, P.M., Ph.D., M.D., Cronin, K.A., Ph.D., Howlader, N., M.S., Berg, C.D., M.D., Chlebowski, R.T., M.D., Ph.D., Feur, E.J., Ph.D., ...Berry, D.A., Ph.D. The Decrease in Breast-Cancer Incidence in 2003 in the United States. The New England Journal of Medicine. 2007. 356. (16).1670-1674.

Jones,M.E., Schoemaker, M.J., Wright, L.,McFadden, E.,Griffin, J.,Thomas,D.,... Swerdlow, A.J. Menopausal hormone therapy and breast cancer: what is the true size of the increased risk? British Journal of Cancer. 2016. 115. (5). 607-615.

Wang, K., Li, F., Chen, L., Lai, Y.M., Xiang Zhang, X., Li, H.Y. Change in risk of breast cancer after receiving hormone replacement therapy by considering effect-modifiers: a systematic review and dose-response meta-analysis of prospective studies. Oncotarget. 2017. 8. (6). 81108-81124.

Kim, S., Ko, Y., Lee, H., Lim, J.E. Menopausal hormone therapy and the risk of breast cancer by histological type and race: a meta-analysis of randomized controlled trials and cohort studies. Breast Cancer Research and Treatment. 2018. 170. (3). 667-675.

Chien, L.N., Huang, Y.J., Shao, Y.H.J., Chang, C.J., Chuang, M.T.,Chiou, H.Y., Yen, Y. Proton pump inhibitors and risk of periampullary cancers—A nested case–control study. International Journal of Cancer. 2015. 138. (206). 1401-1409.

Joe Graedon. (2008). Do Prescription Drugs Cause Cancer? The People's Pharmacy. Retrieved from. https://www.peoplespharmacy.com/2008/10/20/do-prescription-1/

How does chemotherapy affect the risk of second cancers? The American Cancer Society. Retrieved from. https://www.cancer.org/treatment/treatments-and-side-effects/ physical-side-effects/second-cancers-in-adults/chemotherapy.html

Kaldor, J.M., Day, N.E.,Pettersson, F., Clarke, E.A., Pedersen, D.,Mehnert, W.,... Bell, J. Leukemia Following Chemotherapy for Ovarian Cancer. *The New England Journal of Medicine*. 1990. 322. 1-6.

Pastan, I., & Gottesman, M. Multiple-Drug Resistance in Human Cancer. *The New England Journal of Medicine*. 1987. 316. 1388-1393.

Tamargo, J.,, Caballero, R., Delpón, E. Cancer chemotherapy and cardiac arrhythmias: a review. *Drug Safety*. 2015. 38. (2). 129-52.

Pai, V.B., Nahata, M.C., Cardiotoxicity of chemotherapeutic agents: incidence, treatment and prevention. *Drug Safety*. 2000. 22. (4). 263-302.

Newman, T.B.,Hulley, B. (1996). Carcinogenicity of Lipid-Lowering Drugs. *The Journal of the American Medical Association*. 275. (1). 55-60.

Radiation Health Effects, United States Environmental Protection Agency. Retrieved from. https://www.epa.gov/radiation/radiation-health-effects#self

How ionising radiation damages DNA and causes cancer: Two characteristic patterns of DNA damage found. (2016). Wellcome Trust Sanger Institute. Retrieved from. https://www.sanger.ac.uk/news/view/how-ionising-radiation-damages-dna-and-causes-cancer

Sam Behjati, S., Gundem, G., Wedge, D.C., Roberts, N.D., Tarpey, P.S., Cooke, S. L., ...Butler, A.P. Mutational signatures of ionizing radiation in second malignancies. *Nature Communications.* 2016. 7. 12605.

de Martel, C., Ferlay, J., Franceschi, S., Vignat, J., Bray, F., Forman, D., Plumme, M. Global burden of cancers attributable to infections in 2008: a review and synthetic analysis. The Lancet, Oncology. 2012. 13. (6). 607-15.

De Flora, S., & La Maestra, S., Epidemiology of cancers of infectious origin and prevention strategies. *Journal of Preventive Medicine and Hygiene.* 2015. 56. (1). E15-E20.

Moore, P.S., & Chang, Y. Why do viruses cause cancer? Highlights of the first century of human tumour virology. *Nature Reviews Cancer.* 2010. 10. (12). 878-889.

Brindley,P.J., Correia da Costa, J.M., and Sripa, B. Why does infection with some helminths cause cancer? *Trends in Cancer.* 2015. 1. (3). 174-182.

Cohen, L., Sood, A.K., Prinsloo, S., Chaoul, A., (2014). Stress and Tumor Biology: Insights Into Managing Stress to Help Improve Cancer Care. The ASCO Post. Retrieved from. http://www.ascopost.com/issues/january-15-2014/stress-and-tumor-biology-insights-into-managing-stress-to-help-improve-cancer-care/

Moreno-Smith, M., Lutgendorf, S.K., & Sood, A.K. Impact of stress on cancer metastasis. *Future Oncology.* 2010. 6. (12). 1863-1881.

Thaker, P.H., & Sood, A.K. The Neuroendocrine Impact of Chronic Stress on Cancer. *Seminars in Cancer Biology.* 2008. 18. (3). 164-170.

Anil K. Sood, A.K., Lutgendorf, S.K., Stress Influences on Anoikis. *Cancer Prevention Research*. 2011. 4.(4). 481-485.

Baltrusch, H.J., Stangel, W., Titze, I., Stress, cancer and immunity. New developments in biopsychosocial and psychoneuroimmunologic research. *Acta Neurologica (Napoli)*. 1991. 13. (4). 315-27.

Nagaraja, A.S., Armaiz-Pena, G.N., Lutgendorf, S.K., and Sood, A.K., Why stress is BAD for cancer patients. *The Journal of Clinical Investigation*. 2013. 123. (2). 558-560.

Pollak, M.N., Schernhammer, E.S., & Hankinson, S.E., Insulin-like growth factors and neoplasia. *Nature Reviews Cancer*. 2004. 4. 505-518.

Giovannucci, E., Insulin, Insulin-Like Growth Factors and Colon Cancer: A Review of the Evidence. *The Journal of Nutrition*. 12001. 31. (11). 3109S-3120S.

Jiang,Y., Pan, Y., Rhea, P.R., Tan, L., Gagea, M.,Cohen, L.,...Yang, P., A Sucrose-Enriched Diet Promotes Tumorigenesis in Mammary Gland in Part through the 12-Lipoxygenase Pathway. *Cancer Research*. 2016. 76. (1). 24-29.

Peeters, K., Van Leemputte, F., Fischer, B., Bonini, B.M., Quezada, H.,Tsytlonok, M.,... Johan M. Thevelein, J.M., Fructose-1,6-bisphosphate couples glycolytic flux to activation of Ras. *Nature Communications*. 2017. 8. 922.

Tasevska, N.,Jiao, L., Cross, A.J., Kipnis, V., Subar, A.F., Hollenbeck, A.,... Potischman, N., Sugars in diet and risk of cancer in the NIH-AARP Diet and Health Study. *International Journal of Cancer*. 2012. 130. (1). 159-169.

Michaud, DS1., Liu, S., Giovannucci, E., Willett, W.C., Colditz. G.A., Fuchs, C.S., Dietary sugar, glycemic load, and pancreatic cancer risk in a prospective study. *Journal of the National Cancer Institute*. 2002. 94. (17).1293-300.

Larsson, S.C., Bergkvist, L., Wolk, A., Consumption of sugar and sugar-sweetened foods and the risk of pancreatic cancer in a prospective study. *The American Journal of Clinical Nutrition.* 2006. 84. (5). 1171–1176.

Darby, S., Hill, D., Auvinen, A., Barros-Dios, J.M., Baysson, H., Bochicchio, F.,...Doll, R., Radon in homes and risk of lung cancer: collaborative analysis of individual data from 13 European case-control studies. *The BMJ.* 2005. 330. 223.

Torres-Durán, M., Ruano-Ravina, A., Parente-Lamelas, I., Leiro-Fernández, V., Abal-Arca, J., Montero-Martínez, C., Residential radon and lung cancer characteristics in never smokers. *International Journal of Radiation Biology.* 2015. 91. (8). 605-10.

Krewski, D., Lubin, J. H., Zielinski, J.M., Alavanja, M., Catalan, V.S., Field, R.W., ...Homer B., Residential Radon and Risk of Lung Cancer: A Combined Analysis of 7 North American Case-Control Studies. *Epidemiology.* 2005. 16. (2). 137-145.

Lantz, P.M., Mendez, D., & Philbert, M.A., Radon, Smoking, and Lung Cancer: The Need to Refocus Radon Control Policy. *American Journal Public Health.* 2013. 103. (3). 443-447.

Chapter 2: How Cancer can be Prevented

K.L. Bassil, et al. Cancer health effects of pesticides, a Systematic review, *Can Fam Physician.* 2007 Oct; 53(10): 1704–1711.

Minlu Zhang, et al. Body mass index, waist-to-hip ratio and late outcomes: a report from the Shanghai Breast Cancer Survival Study, *Sci Rep.* 2017; 7: 6996.

Zhang C, et al. Maternal obesity and longitudinal ultrasonographic measures of fetal growth: findings from the NICHD fetal growth studies — singletons. *JAMA Pediatrics* 2017

Domenica Rea, et al. Microbiota effects on cancer: from risks to therapies, *Oncotarget.* 2018 Apr 3; 9(25): 17915–17927.

Collaborative Group on Hormonal Factors in Breast Cancer. Breast cancer and breastfeeding. *Lancet.* 2002 Jul 20;360(9328):187-95.

Praud, et al. Cancer incidence and mortality attributable to alcohol consumption, *International Journal of Cancer.* 2016 Mar 15;138(6):1380-7.

Soundararajan, P and Kim, JS. Anti-Carcinogenic Glucosinolates in Cruciferous Vegetables and Their Antagonistic Effects on Prevention of Cancers. *Molecules.* 2018 Nov 15;23(11)

Sood AK and Lutgendorf SK. Stress influences on anoikis. *Cancer Prev Res (Phila).* 2011 Apr;4(4):481-5.

Almendros I and Gozal D. Intermittent hypoxia and cancer: Undesirable bed partners? *Respir Physiol Neurobiol.* 2018 Oct;256:79-86.

Brown JC, Winters-Stone K, Lee A, and Schmitz KH. Cancer, physical activity, and exercise. *Compr Physiol.* 2012 Oct;2(4):2775-809.

Devi KS, Maiti TK. Immunomodulatory and Anti-cancer Properties of Pharmacologically Relevant Mushroom Glycans. *Recent Pat Biotechnol.* 2016;10(1):72-78.

Suresh Bugide and Radoslav Janostiak, Narendra Wajapeyee. Epigenetic Mechanisms Dictating Eradication of Cancer by Natural Killer Cells. *Cancer Review,* vol 4, issue 8, P553-566, AUGUST 01, 2018

Amy Joy Lanou and Barbara Svenson. Reduced cancer risk in vegetarians: an analysis of recent reports. *Cancer Manag Res.* 2011; 3: 1–8.

de Martel C.et al. Global burden of cancers attributable to infections in 2008: a review and synthetic analysis. *Lancet Oncol.* 2012; 13: 607-615

Ahn J.et al. Human gut microbiome and risk for colorectal cancer. *J. Natl. Cancer Inst.* 2013; 105: 1907-1911

Sobhani I.et al. Microbial dysbiosis in colorectal cancer (CRC) patients. *PLoS ONE.* 2011; 6: e16393

Nelson DE, Jarman DW, Rehm J, et al. Alcohol-attributable cancer deaths and years of potential life lost in the United States. *American Journal of Public Health.* 2013;103(4):641-648.

LoConte NK, Brewster AM, Kaur JS, Merrill JK, Alberg AJ. Alcohol and cancer: A statement of the American Society of Clinical Oncology. *Journal of Clinical Oncology.* 2018; 36(1):83-93.

Crusz S.M.Balkwill F.R. Inflammation and cancer: advances and new agents. *Nat. Rev. Clin.* Oncol. 2015

Elinav E.et al. Inflammation-induced cancer: crosstalk between tumours, immune cells and microorganisms. *Nat. Rev. Cancer.* 2013; 13: 759-771

Morvan M.G.Lanier L.L. NK cells and cancer: you can teach innate cells new tricks. *Nat. Rev. Cancer.* 2016; 16: 7-19

Ben-Eliyahu S.et al. Acute alcohol intoxication suppresses natural killer cell activity and promotes tumor metastasis. *Nat. Med.* 1996; 2: 457-460

Guillerey C.et al. Targeting natural killer cells in cancer immunotherapy. *Nat. Immunol.* 2016; 17: 1025-1036

Chapter 3
How is Cancer Diagnosed?

Kwapisz, D., The first liquid biopsy test approved. Is it a new era of mutation testing for non-small cell lung cancer? Annals of Translational Medicine. 2017. 5. (3). 46.

Single Blood Test Screens for Eight Cancer Type : Provides unique new framework for early detection of the most common cancers. (2018). Johns Hopkins Kimmel Cancer Center. Retrieved from.
https://www.hopkinsmedicine.org/news/newsroom/news-releases/
single-blood-test-screens-for-eight-cancer-types

Rahman, N., Mainstreaming genetic testing of cancer predisposition genes. Clinical Medicine (London). 2014. 14. (4). 436-439;

Timon Hussain, T., & Nguyen, Q.T., Molecular Imaging for Cancer Diagnosis and Surgery. *Advanced Drug Delivery Reviews.* 2014. 66. 90-100.

FDA approves first blood test to detect gene mutation associated with non-small cell lung cancer. (2016). U.S. Food and Drug Administration. Retrieved from.
https://www.fda.gov/NewsEvents/Newsroom/PressAnnouncements/
ucm504488.htm

Tsai V.W., Macia, L., Johnen, H,, Kuffner, T., Manadhar, R., Jørgensen, S.B., Lin, S., TGF-b superfamily cytokine MIC-1/GDF15 is a physiological appetite and body weight regulator. *PloS One.* 2013. 8.(2). E55174.

When is Weight Loss a Sign of Cancer? (2017). Insight from Dana-Farber Cancer Institute. Retrieved from.
https://blog.dana-farber.org/insight/2017/06/when-is-weight-loss-a-sign-of-cancer/

Nagpal, M., Singh, S.,Singh, P., Chauhan, P., and Zaidi, M.A., Tumor markers: A diagnostic tool. *National Journal of Maxillofacial Surgery.* 2016. 7. (1). 17-20.

Tumor Markers. National Cancer Institute. Retrieved from.
https://www.cancer.gov/about-cancer/diagnosis-staging/diagnosis/
tumor-markers-fact-sheet

Signs and Symptoms of Endometrial Cancer. American Cancer Society. Retrieved from. https://www.cancer.org/cancer/endometrial-cancer/detection-diagnosis-staging/signs-and-symptoms.html

Signs and Symptoms of Colorectal Cancer. American Cancer Society. Retrieved from. https://www.cancer.org/latest-news/signs-and-symptoms-of-colon-cancer.html

Signs and Symptoms of Lung Cancer. American Cancer Society. Retrieved from. https://www.cancer.org/cancer/lung-cancer/prevention-and-early-detection/signs-and-symptoms.html

When is Weight Loss a Sign of Cancer? (2017). Insight from Dana-Farber Cancer Institute. Retrieved from. https://blog.dana-farber.org/insight/2017/06/when-is-weight-loss-a-sign-of-cancer/

Symptoms of Cancer. National Institute of Cancer. Retrieved from. https://www.cancer.gov/about-cancer/diagnosis-staging/symptoms

Causes of Sweating. Cancer Research UK. Retrieved from. https://www.cancerresearchuk.org/about-cancer/coping/physically/skin-problems/dealing-with-sweating/causes

What's the Connection Between Night Sweats and Cancer. (2016). Insight from Dana-Farber Cancer Institute. Retrieved from. https://blog.dana-farber.org/insight/2016/09/whats-the-connection-between-night-sweats-and-cancer/

Singh, G.K., Yadav, V., Singh, P., and Bhowmik, K.T., Radiation-Induced Malignancies Making Radiotherapy a "Two-Edged Sword": A Review of Literature. *World Journal of Oncology*. 2017. 8. (1). 1-6.

Braunstein, S., & Nakamura, J.L., Radiotherapy-Induced Malignancies: Review of Clinical Features, Pathobiology, and Evolving Approaches for Mitigating Risk. *Frontiers in Oncology*. 2013. 3. 73.

Chapter 4
Integrative Cancer Care with Chinese Medicine

Zia FZ. Olaku O. Bao T. et al. The National Cancer Institute's Conference on Acupuncture for Symptom Management in Oncology: State of the Science, Evidence, and Research Gaps. *JNCI Monographs*, 2017. 52:1.

Chien TJ. Liu CY. and Hsu CH. Integrating Acupuncture into Cancer Care. *J Tradit Complement Med*. 2013. 3(4): 234–239.

Asadpour R. Meng Z. Kessel K.K. and Combs S.E. Use of acupuncture to alleviate side effects in radiation oncology: Current evidence and future directions. *Adv Radiat Oncol*. 2016 Oct-Dec. 1(4): 344–350.

Garcia MK. McQuade J. Haddad R. et al. Systematic Review of Acupuncture in Cancer Care: A Synthesis of the Evidence. *J Clin Oncol*. 2013 Mar 1; 31(7): 952–960

Li X. Yang G. Li X. et al. Traditional Chinese medicine in cancer care: a review of controlled clinical studies published in Chinese. *PLoS One*. 2013;8(4):e60338.

Ye L. Jia Y. Ji K. et al. Traditional Chinese medicine in the prevention and treatment of cancer and cancer metastasis. *Oncol Lett*. 2015 Sep; 10(3): 1240–1250.

Lu W. Dean-Clower E. Doherty-Gilman A. and Rosenthal DS. The Value of Acupuncture in Cancer Care. *Hematol Oncol Clin North Am*. 2008 Aug; 22(4): 631–viii.

Ling Y. Traditional Chinese medicine in the treatment of symptoms in patients with advanced cancer. *Ann Palliat Med*. 2013 Jul;2(3):141-52.

Liu J. Wang S. Zhang Y. Fan HT. and Lin HS. Traditional Chinese medicine and cancer: History, present situation, and development. *Thorac Cancer.* 2015 Sep; 6(5): 561–569.

Jia L., Lin H., Oppenheim J., et al. US National Cancer Institute–China Collaborative Studies on Chinese Medicine and Cancer. *JNCI Monographs*, Volume 2017, Issue 52, 1 November 2017, lgx007.

Chung VC. et al., Chinese Herbal Medicine for Symptom Management in Cancer Palliative Care: Systematic Review And Meta-analysis. *Medicine (Baltimore).* 2016 Feb; 95(7): e2793.

Baumann S., et al. Wogonin preferentially kills malignant lymphocytes and suppresses T-cell tumor growth by inducing PLCgamma1- and Ca2+-dependent apoptosis. *Blood.* 2008 Feb 15;111(4):2354-63. Epub 2007 Dec 10.

Jiao L., et al. Effects of Chinese Medicine as Adjunct Medication for Adjuvant Chemotherapy Treatments of Non-Small Cell Lung Cancer Patients. *Sci Rep.* 2017; 7: 46524

Ma L., et al. Acupuncture as a complementary therapy in chemotherapy-induced nausea and vomiting. *Proc (Bayl Univ Med Cent).* 2009 Apr; 22(2): 138–141.

Shen J., et. al. Electroacupuncture for control of myeloablative chemotherapy-induced emesis: A randomized controlled trial. JAMA. 2000 Dec 6;284(21):2755-61.

Zhou J., et al. The effect of acupuncture on chemotherapy-associated gastrointestinal symptoms in gastric cancer. *Curr Oncol.* 2017 Feb; 24(1):e1–e5.

Mustian KM., et al. Treatment of Nausea and Vomiting During Chemotherapy. *US Oncol Hematol.* 2011; 7(2): 91–97.

Rithirangsriroj K. Manchana T., and Akkayagorn L. Efficacy of acupuncture in prevention of delayed chemotherapy induced nausea and vomiting in gynecologic cancer patients. *Gynecol Oncol.* 2015 Jan;136(1):82-6.

Collins K B. and Thomas D J. Acupuncture and acupressure for the management of chemotherapy-induced nausea and vomiting. *J Am Acad Nurse Pract.* 2004 Feb;16(2):76-80.

Ling Y. Traditional Chinese medicine in the treatment of symptoms in patients with advanced cancer. *Ann Palliat Med.* 2013 Jul;2(3):141-52.

Janelsins M C., et al., Current Pharmacotherapy for Chemotherapy-Induced Nausea and Vomiting in Cancer Patients. *Expert Opin Pharmacother.* 2013 Apr; 14(6): 757–766.

Nasir S.S., and Schwartzberg L.S. Recent Advances in Preventing Chemotherapy-Induced Nausea and Vomiting. 2016. Retrieved from. https://www.cancernetwork.com/authors/lee-s-schwartzberg-md

Chen CM. Lin LZ. and Zhang EX. Standardized treatment of chinese medicine decoction for cancer pain patients with opioid-induced constipation: A multi-center prospective randomized controlled study. Chin J Integr Med. 2014 Jul;20(7):496-502.

Qi FH, Li AY, Inagaki Y, et al. Chinese herbal medicines as adjuvant treatment during chemo- or radio-therapy for cancer. *BioScience Trends.* 2010 ;4(6):297-307.

McQuade RM. Stojanovska V. Abalo R. et al. Chemotherapy-Induced Constipation and Diarrhea: Pathophysiology, Current and Emerging Treatments. Front Pharmacol. 2016; 7: 414.

Hsu PY. Yang SH. Tsang NM. et al. Efficacy of Traditional Chinese Medicine in Xerostomia and Quality of Life during Radiotherapy for Head and Neck Cancer: A Prospective Pilot Study. *Evid Based Complement Alternat Med.* 2016; 2016: 8359251.

Park B. Noh H. and Choi DJ. Herbal Medicine for Xerostomia in Cancer Patients: A Systematic Review of Randomized Controlled Trials. *Integr Cancer Ther*. 2018 Jun; 17(2): 179–191.

George SJ. What is the role of acupuncture in the treatment of oncology patients with xerostomia? *Australian Journal of Acupuncture and Chinese Medicine*. 11(1); 2017.

Meng Z. Garcia MK. and Hu C. Randomized controlled trial of acupuncture for prevention of radiation-induced xerostomia among patients with nasopharyngeal carcinoma. *Cancer*. 2012 Jul 1; 118(13): 3337–3344.

Acupuncture Eases Radiation-induced Dry Mouth In Cancer Patients. University of Texas M. D. Anderson Cancer Center. April 25, 2009. Retrieved from. https://www.sciencedaily.com/releases/2009/04/090420151232.htm

Blom M. Dawidson I. Fernberg J-O. Johnson G. and Angmar-Månsson B. Acupuncture treatment of patients with radiation-induced xerostomia. *European Journal of Cancer Part B: Oral Oncology*. 1996. 32(3): Pages 182-190.

Homba KA. Wu H. Tarima S. and Wang D. Improvement of radiation-induced xerostomia with acupuncture: A retrospective analysis. *Acupuncture and Related Therapies*. 2014. 2(2):34-38.

Johnstone PAS. Peng P. and May BC. Acupuncture for pilocarpine-resistant xerostomia following radiotherapy for head and neck malignancies. *International Journal of Radiation Oncology*Biology*Physics*. 2001. 50 (2):353-357.

Wong RKW. Jones GW. Sagar SM. et al. A Phase I–II study in the use of acupuncture-like transcutaneous nerve stimulation in the treatment of radiation-induced xerostomia in head-and-neck cancer patients treated with radical radiotherapy. *International Journal of Radiation Oncology*Biology*Physics*. 2003. 57(2):472-480.

Zhuang L. Yang Z. Zeng X. et al. The preventive and therapeutic effect of acupuncture for radiation-induced xerostomia in patients with head and neck cancer: a systematic review. *Integr Cancer Ther.* 2013 May;12(3): 197-205.

Javdan B. and Cassileth B. Acupuncture Research at Memorial Sloan Kettering Cancer Center. *J Acupunct Meridian Stud.* 2015 Jun;8(3):115-21.

Blom M. Dawidson I. and Angmar-Månsson B. The effect of acupuncture on salivary flow rates in patients with xerostomia. *Oral Surgery, Oral Medicine, Oral Pathology, Oral Radiology.* 1992. 73(3): 293-298.

Cho JH. Chung WK. Kang W. et al. Manual acupuncture improved quality of life in cancer patients with radiation-induced xerostomia. *J Altern Complement Med.* 2008 Jun;14(5):523-6.

Wang T. Deng R. Tan JY. and Guan FG. Acupoints Stimulation for Anxiety and Depression in Cancer Patients: A Quantitative Synthesis of Randomized Controlled Trials. *Evid Based Complement Alternat Med.* 2016; 2016: 5645632.

Acupuncture in the Treatment of Cancer-Related Psychological Symptoms Haddad NE. and Palesh O., Acupuncture in the Treatment of Cancer-Related Psychological Symptoms. *Integrative Cancer Therapies* 2014, Vol. 13(5) 371 –385

Lu W. and Rosenthal DS. Acupuncture for Cancer Pain and Related Symptoms. *Curr Pain Headache Rep.* 2013 Mar; 17(3): 321.

Hu C. Zhang H. Wu W. et al. Acupuncture for Pain Management in Cancer: A Systematic Review and Meta-Analysis. *Evid Based Complement Alternat Med.* 2016; 2016: 1720239.

Oh B. et al. Acupuncture for treatment of arthralgia secondary to aromatase inhibitor therapy in women with early breast cancer: pilot study. *Acupunct Med.* 2013 Sep;31(3):264-71.

Patel J. et al. Efficacy of Acupuncture (ACU) Therapy for Cancer-Related Pain Management in Oncology Patients (Pts) (S729). Journal of Pain and Symptom Management. 2016. 51(2). 422–423.

Vinjamury SP. et al. Effects of acupuncture for cancer pain and quality of life – a case series. Chin Med. 2013; 8: 15.

Peiwen Li. Management of Cancer with Chinese Medicine. UK. Donica Publishing Ltd. 2003.

Lahans Tai. Integrating Conventional and Chinese Medicine in Cancer Care. Philadelphia, PA. Churchill Livingstone Elsevier. 2007.

Trian Niko. Chinese Medicine in Cancer Care. San Bernardino, CA. Create Space An Amazon.com Company. 2016.

Chapter 5:
What You Eat - Diet, Nutrition, and Supplements

Food and Cancer Risk. ASCO. Retrieved from.
https://www.cancer.net/navigating-cancer-care/prevention-and-healthy-living/food-and-cancer-risk

Alcohol. ASCO. Retrieved from.
https://www.cancer.net/navigating-cancer-care/prevention-and-healthy-living/alcohol

Leischner C. et al. Nutritional immunology: function of natural killer cells and their modulation by resveratrol for cancer prevention and treatment. Nutr J. 2016 May 4;15(1):47.

Leoncini E. Carotenoid Intake from Natural Sources and Head and Neck Cancer: A Systematic Review and Meta-analysis of Epidemiological Studies. 2015. DOI: 10.1158/1055-9965.EPI-15-0053.

Tocaciu S. et al. The Effect of Undaria pinnatifida Fucoidan on the Pharmacokinetics of Letrozole and Tamoxifen in Patients With Breast Cancer. *Integr Cancer Ther.* 2018 Mar; 17(1): 99–105.

Ikeguchi M. et al. Fucoidan reduces the toxicities of chemotherapy for patients with unresectable advanced or recurrent colorectal cancer. *Oncol Lett.* 2011 Mar;2(2):319-322.

Takahashi H. et al. An Exploratory Study on the Anti-inflammatory Effects of Fucoidan in Relation to Quality of Life in Advanced Cancer Patients. *Integr Cancer Ther.* 2018 Jun;17(2):282-291.

Atashrazm F. et al. Fucoidan and Cancer: A Multifunctional Molecule with Anti-Tumor Potential. *Mar Drugs.* 2015 Apr; 13(4): 2327–2346.

Ale MT. et al. Fucoidan from Sargassum sp. and Fucus vesiculosus reduces cell viability of lung carcinoma and melanoma cells in vitro and activates natural killer cells in mice in vivo. *Int J Biol Macromol.* 2011 Oct 1;49(3):331-6.

Lee H. Kim JS. and Kim E., Fucoidan from seaweed Fucus vesiculosus inhibits migration and invasion of human lung cancer cell via PI3K-Akt-mTOR pathways. *PLoS One.* 2012;7(11):e50624.

Shukla S. Meeran SM. and Katiyar SK. Epigenetic regulation by selected dietary phytochemicals in cancer chemoprevention. *Cancer Lett.* 2014 Dec 1;355(1):9-17.

Funk K. Breasts: The Owner's Manual: every woman's guide to reducing cancer risk, making treatment choices, and optimizing outcomes. Nashville, Tennessee. W Publishing. 2018.

Greger M. and Stone G. How Not to Die, Discover the Foods Scientifically Proven to Prevent and Reverse Disease. New York, New York. Flatiron Books. 2015.

Wu AH. Lee E. and Vigen C. Soy isoflavones and breast cancer. Am Soc Clin Oncol Educ Book. 2013:102-6.

Xiao Ou Shu. et al. Soy Food Intake and Breast Cancer Survival. JAMA. 2009 Dec 9; 302(22): 2437–2443.
Mueller SO. Phytoestrogens and their human metabolites show distinct agonistic and antagonistic properties on estrogen receptor alpha (ERalpha) and ERbeta in human cells. *Toxicol Sci.* 2004 Jul;80(1):14-25.

Oseni T. et al. Selective estrogen receptor modulators and phytoestrogens. *Planta Med.* 2008 Oct;74(13):1656-65.

Ziaei S. and Halaby R. Dietary Isoflavones and Breast Cancer Risk. *Medicines (Basel).* 2017 Jun; 4(2): 18.

Guha N. Soy isoflavones and risk of cancer recurrence in a cohort of breast cancer survivors: the Life After Cancer Epidemiology study. *Breast Cancer Res Treat.* 2009 Nov;118(2):395-405.

Kristo AS. Klimis-Zacas D. and Sikalidis AK. Protective Role of Dietary Berries in Cancer. *Antioxidants (Basel).* 2016 Dec; 5(4): 37.

Baby B. Antony P. Vijayan R. Antioxidant and anticancer properties of berries. *Crit Rev Food Sci Nutr.* 2017 Jun 13:1-17.

Davidson KT. et al. Beyond Conventional Medicine - a Look at Blueberry, a Cancer-Fighting Superfruit. *Pathol Oncol Res.* 2018 Oct;24(4):733-738.

Wang E. Antiproliferative and proapoptotic activities of anthocyanin and anthocyanidin extracts from blueberry fruits on B16-F10 melanoma cells. *Food Nutr Res.* 2017 Jun 19;61(1)

Johnson SA. Arjmandi BH. Evidence for anti-cancer properties of blueberries: a mini-review. *Anticancer Agents Med Chem.* 2013 Oct;13(8):1142-8.

Zhang HM. et al. Research progress on the anticarcinogenic actions and mechanisms of ellagic acid. *Cancer Biol Med.* 2014 Jun; 11(2): 92–100.

Liu Q. et al. Ellagic acid promotes A549 cell apoptosis via regulating the phosphoinositide 3-kinase/protein kinase B pathway. *Exp Ther Med.* 2018 Jul; 16(1): 347–352.

Ceci C. et al. Experimental Evidence of the Antitumor, Antimetastatic and Antiangiogenic Activity of Ellagic Acid. *Nutrients.* 2018 Nov; 10(11): 1756.

Cheng H. Ellagic acid inhibits the proliferation of human pancreatic carcinoma PANC-1 cells in vitro and in vivo. *Oncotarget.* 2017 Feb 14; 8(7): 12301–12310.

Royston KJ. and Tollefsbol TO. The Epigenetic Impact of Cruciferous Vegetables on Cancer Prevention. *Curr Pharmacol Rep.* 2015 Feb 1; 1(1): 46–51.

Murillo G. and Mehta RG. Cruciferous vegetables and cancer prevention. *Nutr Cancer.* 2001;41(1-2):17-28.

Servan-Schreiber, D. Anticancer: A New Way of Life. New York, NY. Penguin Books. 2017.

Khayat, D. The Anti-Cancer Diet. New York, NY. W.W. Norton & Company, Inc. 2010.

Campbell, TT. and Campbell TM. The China Study. Dallax, TX. BenBella Books. 2016.

Beliveau R. and Gingras D. Foods to Fight Cancer. New York, NY. DK Publishing. 2017.

Quillin P. and Quillin N. Beating Cancer with Nutrition. Carlsbad, CA. Nutrition Times Press. 2005.

Jahanbani R. Antioxidant and Anticancer Activities of Walnut (Juglans regia L.) Protein Hydrolysates Using Different Proteases. *Plant Foods Hum Nutr.* 2016 Dec;71(4):402-409.

Falasca M. Casari I. and Maffucci T. Cancer Chemoprevention With Nuts. *JNCI: Journal of the National Cancer Institute.* 106.(9). 1 September 2014, dju238,

Calado A. et al. The Effect of Flaxseed in Breast Cancer: A Literature Review. *Front Nutr.* 2018; 5: 4.

Demark-Wahnefried W. et al. Flaxseed supplementation (not dietary fat restriction) reduces prostate cancer proliferation rates in men pre-surgery. *Cancer Epidemiol Biomarkers Prev.* 2008 Dec;17(12):3577-87.

Sengupta A. Ghosh S. and Bhattacharjee S. Allium vegetables in cancer prevention: an overview. *Asian Pac J Cancer Prev.* 2004 Jul-Sep;5(3):237-45.

Nicastro HL. Ross SA. and Milner JA. Garlic and onions: their cancer prevention properties. *Cancer Prev Res (Phila).* 2015 Mar;8(3):181-9.

Galeone C. et al. Onion and garlic use and human cancer. *Am J Clin Nutr.* 2006 Nov;84(5):1027-32.

Luo WP. et al. High consumption of vegetable and fruit colour groups is inversely associated with the risk of colorectal cancer: a case-control study. *Br J Nutr.* 2015 Apr 14;113(7):1129-38

Christensen KY. et al. The risk of lung cancer related to dietary intake of flavonoids. *Nutr Cancer.* 2012;64(7):964-74

Li WQ. et al. Citrus consumption and cancer incidence: the Ohsaki cohort study. *Int J Cancer.* 2010 Oct 15;127(8):1913-22.

Zhao W. Liu L. and Xu S. Intakes of citrus fruit and risk of esophageal cancer: A meta-analysis. *Medicine (Baltimore).* 2018 Mar;97(13):e0018.

Bae JM. Lee EJ. and Guyatt G. Citrus fruit intake and stomach cancer risk: a quantitative systematic review. *Gastric Cancer.* 2008;11(1):23-32.

Cirmi S. et al. Chemopreventive Agents and Inhibitors of Cancer Hallmarks: May Citrus Offer New Perspectives? *Nutrients.* 2016 Nov; 8(11): 698.

Sharma P. Sarah F. McClees SF. and Afaq F. Pomegranate for Prevention and Treatment of Cancer: An Update. *Molecules.* 2017 Jan 24; 22(1): E177.

Panth N. Manandhar B. and Paudel KR. Anticancer Activity of Punica granatum (Pomegranate): A Review. *Phytother Res.* 2017 Apr;31(4): 568-578.

Lee Y. Cancer Chemopreventive Potential of Procyanidin. *Toxicol Res.* 2017 Oct; 33(4): 273–282.

Delphi L. et al. Pectic-Oligoshaccharides from Apples Induce Apoptosis and Cell Cycle Arrest in MDA-MB-231 Cells, a Model of Human Breast Cancer. *Asian Pac J Cancer Prev.* 2015;16(13):5265-71.

Li S. et al. Quercetin enhances chemotherapeutic effect of doxorubicin against human breast cancer cells while reducing toxic side effects of it. *Biomedicine & Pharmacotherapy.* 2018. 100. 441-447.

Fabiani R. Minelli L. and Rosignoli P. Apple intake and cancer risk: a systematic review and meta-analysis of observational studies. *Public Health Nutr.* 2016 Oct;19(14):2603-17

Zhang D. et al. Apple polysaccharides induce apoptosis in colorectal cancer cells. *Int J Mol Med.* 2012 Jul;30(1):100-6.

He X. and Liu RH. Triterpenoids Isolated from Apple Peels Have Potent Antiproliferative Activity and May Be Partially Responsible for Apple's Anticancer Activity. J. Agric. *Food Chem.*, 2007, 55 (11), pp 4366–4370.

Sangaramoorthy M. Koo J. and John EM. Intake of bean fiber, beans, and grains and reduced risk of hormone receptor-negative breast cancer: the San Francisco Bay Area Breast Cancer Study. *Cancer Med.* 2018 May; 7(5): 2131–2144.

Mudryj AN. Yu N. and Aukema HM. Nutritional and health benefits of pulses. *Appl Physiol Nutr Metab.* 2014 Nov;39(11):1197-204.

Kumar Ganesan K. and Xu B. Polyphenol-Rich Lentils and Their Health Promoting Effects. Int J Mol Sci. 2017 Nov; 18(11): 2390.

Li J. and Mao QQ. Legume intake and risk of prostate cancer: a meta-analysis of prospective cohort studies. *Oncotarget.* 2017 Jul 4; 8(27): 44776–44784.

Zhu B. et al. Dietary legume consumption reduces risk of colorectal cancer: evidence from a meta-analysis of cohort studies. *Sci Rep.* 2015; 5: 8797.

Chen P. et al. Lycopene and Risk of Prostate Cancer A Systematic Review and Meta-Analysis. *Medicine (Baltimore).* 2015 Aug; 94(33): e1260.

Vallverdú-Queralt A. et al. Carotenoid Profile of Tomato Sauces: Effect of Cooking Time and Content of Extra Virgin Olive Oil. *Int J Mol Sci.* 2015 May; 16(5): 9588–9599.

Palozza P. et al. Tomato Lycopene and Lung Cancer Prevention: From Experimental to Human Studies. *Cancers (Basel).* 2011 Jun; 3(2): 2333–2357.

Kim MJ. and Kim H. Anticancer Effect of Lycopene in Gastric Carcinogenesis. *J Cancer Prev.* 2015 Jun; 20(2): 92–96.

Zheng J. et al. Spices for Prevention and Treatment of Cancers. *Nutrients.* 2016 Aug; 8(8): 495.

Li H. et al. Capsaicin and Piperine Can Overcome Multidrug Resistance in Cancer Cells to Doxorubicin. *Molecules.* 2018 Mar 2;23(3).

Dutta A. and Chakraborty A. Cinnamon in Anticancer Armamentarium: A Molecular Approach. *J Toxicol.* 2018; 2018: 8978731.

Butt MS. et al. Anti-oncogenic perspectives of spices/herbs: A comprehensive review. *EXCLI J.* 2013; 12: 1043–1065.

Muhammad A. et al. Spices with Breast Cancer Chemopreventive and Therapeutic Potentials: A Functional Foods Based-Review. *Anticancer Agents Med Chem.* 2018;18(2):182-194.

Prasad S. and Tyagi AK. Ginger and Its Constituents: Role in Prevention and Treatment of Gastrointestinal Cancer. *Gastroenterol Res Pract.* 2015; 2015: 142979.

Meng B. et al. Anticancer Effects of Gingerol in Retinoblastoma Cancer Cells (RB355 Cell Line) Are Mediated via Apoptosis Induction, Cell Cycle Arrest and Upregulation of PI3K/Akt Signaling Pathway. *Med Sci Monit.* 2018; 24: 1980–1987.

Chapter 6:
What You Do - Exercise, Qi Gong, Meditation and Sleep

Van Vu D. et al. Effects of Qigong on symptom management in cancer patients: A systematic review. *Complement Ther Clin Pract.* 2017 Nov;29: 111-121.

Oh B. et al. A critical review of the effects of medical Qigong on quality of life, immune function, and survival in cancer patients. *Integr Cancer Ther.* 2012 Jun;11(2):101-10.

Larkey LK. et al. Exploratory outcome assessment of Qigong/Tai Chi Easy on Breast cancer survivors. *Complement Ther Med.* 2016 Dec; 29: 196–203.

Lee MS. et al. Qigong for cancer treatment: a systematic review of controlled clinical trials. *Acta Oncol.* 2007;46(6):717-22.

Overcash J. Will KM. and Weisenburger Lipetz D. The Benefits of Medical Qigong in Patients With Cancer: A Descriptive Pilot Study. *CJON 2013*, 17(6), 654-658.

Ott MJ. Norris RL. and Bauer-Wu SM. Mindfulness Meditation for Oncology Patients: A Discussion and Critical Review. *Integrative Cancer Therapies*. 2006. 5(2); 98-108.

Oh B, Butow P, Boyle F, Costa DSJ, Pavlakis N, et al. Effects of Qigong on Quality of Life, Fatigue, Stress, Neuropathy, and Sexual Function in Women with Metastatic Breast Cancer: A Feasibility Study. *Int J Phys Med Rehabil.* 2014. 2:217.

Larkey LK. et al. Randomized Controlled Trial of Qigong/Tai Chi Easy on Cancer-Related Fatigue in Breast Cancer Survivors. *Ann Behav Med.* 2015 Apr; 49(2): 165–176.

Oh B. et al. Impact of Medical Qigong on quality of life, fatigue, mood and inflammation in cancer patients: a randomized controlled trial. *Ann Oncol.* 2010 Mar; 21(3): 608–614.

Zhang MF. et al. Effectiveness of Mindfulness-based Therapy for Reducing Anxiety and Depression in Patients With Cancer A Meta-analysis. *Medicine (Baltimore).* 2015 Nov; 94(45): e0897.

Bower JE. et al. Mindfulness meditation for younger breast cancer survivors: A randomized controlled trial. *Cancer.* 2015 Apr 15; 121(8): 1231–1240.

Sanada K. et al. Effects of mindfulness-based interventions on biomarkers in healthy and cancer populations: a systematic review. *BMC Complement Altern Med.* 2017 Feb 23;17(1):125.

Garland SN. et al. Increased mindfulness is related to improved stress and mood following participation in a mindfulness-based stress reduction program in individuals with cancer. *Integr Cancer Ther.* 2013 Jan;12(1):31-40.

Piet J. Würtzen H. and Zachariae R. The effect of mindfulness-based therapy on symptoms of anxiety and depression in adult cancer patients and survivors: a systematic review and meta-analysis. *J Consult Clin Psychol.* 2012 Dec;80(6):1007-20.

Ciro Conversano C. et al. Optimism and Its Impact on Mental and Physical Well-Being. *Clin Pract Epidemiol Ment Health.* 2010; 6: 25–29.

Würtzen H. et al. Mindfulness significantly reduces self-reported levels of anxiety and depression: results of a randomised controlled trial among 336 Danish women treated for stage I-III breast cancer. *Eur J Cancer.* 2013 Apr;49(6):1365-73.

Johns SA. et al. Randomized controlled pilot trial of mindfulness-based stress reduction for breast and colorectal cancer survivors: effects on cancer-related cognitive impairment. *J Cancer Surviv.* 2016 Jun;10(3):437-48.

Charalambous A. et al. Guided Imagery And Progressive Muscle Relaxation as a Cluster of Symptoms Management Intervention in Patients Receiving Chemotherapy: A Randomized Control Trial. *PLoS One.* 2016; 11(6): e0156911.

Chen SF. et al. Effect of Relaxation With Guided Imagery on The Physical and Psychological Symptoms of Breast Cancer Patients Undergoing Chemotherapy. *Iran Red Crescent Med J.* 2015 Nov; 17(11): e31277.

León-Pizarro C. et al. A randomized trial of the effect of training in relaxation and guided imagery techniques in improving psychological and quality-of-life indices for gynecologic and breast brachytherapy patients. *Psychooncology.* 2007 Nov;16(11):971-9.

Shahriari M. et al. Effects of progressive muscle relaxation, guided imagery and deep diaphragmatic breathing on quality of life in elderly with breast or prostate cancer. *J Educ Health Promot.* 2017; 6: 1.

Oh B. et al. Randomized clinical trial: The Impact of Medical Qigong (traditional Chinese medicine) on fatigue, quality of life, side effects, mood status and inflammation of cancer patients. *Journal of Clinical Oncology* 26, no. 15_suppl (May 20 2008) 9565-9565.

Chapter 7: Who You Are

Reynaert C1, Libert Y, Janne P. Psychogenesis of cancer: between myths, misuses and reality. *Bull Cancer.* 2000 Sep;87(9):655-64.

Grov EK, et al. The personality trait of neuroticism is strongly associated with long-term morbidity in testicular cancer survivors. *Acta Oncol.* 2009;48(6):842-9.

Temoshok L, Heller BW, Sagebiel RW, et al. The relationship of psychosocial factors to prognostic indicators in cutaneous malignant melanoma, *J Psychosom Res.* , 1985, vol. 29 2(pg. 139-153)

Hislop TG, Waxler NE, Coldman AJ, et al. The prognostic significance of psychosocial factors in women with breast cancer, *J Chronic Dis*, 1987, vol. 40 7(pg. 729-735)

Nakaya N, Hansen PE, Schapiro IR, et al. Personality traits and cancer survival: a Danish Cohort Study, *Br J Cancer*, 2006, vol. 95 2(pg. 146-152)

Caryn Aviv, et al. The benefits of prayer on mood and well-being of breast cancer survivors. *Support Care Cancer.* 2009 Mar; 17(3): 295–306.

Eremin O, et al. Immuno-modulatory effects of relaxation training and guided imagery in women with locally advanced breast cancer undergoing multimodality therapy: a randomised controlled trial. *Breast.* 2009 Feb;18(1):17-25.

Fann JR, Ell K, Sharpe M. Resilience in Cancer Patients Front. *Psychiatry*, 05 April 2019

Annina Seiler and Josef Jenewein. Integrating psychosocial care into cancer services. *J Clin Oncol.* 2012 Apr 10; 30(11):1178-86.

Mao Shing Ni. Live Your Ultimate Life: Ancient Wisdom to Harness Success, Health and Happiness. *Tao of Wellness Press.* Jan 2016.

Hajime Iwasa, et al. Personality and All-Cause Mortality Among Older Adults Dwelling in a Japanese Community: A Five-Year Population-Based Prospective Cohort Study. *American J of Geri Psych.* May 2008; 16 (5): 399–405.

Chapter 8: Where You Are

Tasha Stoiber, et al. Applying a cumulative risk framework to drinking water assessment. *Environmental Health,* 2019:18:37

K.L. Bassil, et al. Cancer health effects of pesticides, a systematic review. *Can Fam Physician.* 2007 Oct; 53(10): 1704–1711.

Environmental Working Group. The 2019 Dirty Dozen. https://www.ewg.org/foodnews/summary.php#dirty-dozen

J. Baudry et al., Association of Frequency of Organic Food Consumption with Cancer Risk. *JAMA Internal Medicine,* 2018; 178(12):1597-1606.

Lester MR, Sulfite sensitivity: significance in human health. *J Am Coll Nutr.* 1995 Jun;14(3):229-32.

Peng Song, Lei Wu, and Wenxian Guan. Dietary Nitrates, Nitrites, and Nitrosamines Intake and the Risk of Gastric Cancer: A Meta-Analysis. *Nutrients.* 2015 Dec; 7(12): 9872–9895.

Kobylewski S and Jacobson MF. Toxicology of food dyes. *Int J Occup Environ Health.* 2012 Jul-Sep;18(3):220-46.

Sang-Hee Jeong, et al. Risk Assessment of Growth Hormones and Antimicrobial Residues in Meat. *Toxicol Res.* 2010 Dec; 26(4): 301–313.

Quach T, et al. Adverse birth outcomes and maternal complications in licensed cosmetologists and manicurists in California. *Int Arch Occup Environ Health.* 2015 Oct;88(7):823-33.

National Institute of Environmental Health and Safety. National Toxicology Program. Benzidine and Dyes Metabolized to Benzidine, *Report on Carcinogens, Fourteenth Edition.* Triangle Park, NC: , 2016. Available online. Last accessed January 31, 2019.

Environmental Protection Agency. A Citizen's Guide to Radon. https://www.epa.gov/sites/production/files/2016-12/documents/ 2016_a_citizens_guide_to_radon.pdf

Hauptmann M, Stewart PA, Lubin JH, et al. Mortality from lymphohematopoietic malignancies and brain cancer among embalmers exposed to formaldehyde. *Journal of the National Cancer Institute* 2009; 101(24):1696–1708.

International Agency for Research on Cancer (IARC). Agents Classified by the IARC Monographs, Volumes 1–123. 2019. Accessed at https://monographs.iarc.fr/agents-classified-by-the-iarc/ on March 12, 2019.

International Agency for Research on Cancer. IARC Monographs on the Evaluation of Carcinogenic Risks to Humans. Volume 102, part 2: Non-Ionizing Radiation, Radiofrequency Electromagnetic Fields. 2013. Accessed at http://monographs.iarc.fr/ENG/Monographs/vol102/mono102.pdf on October 15, 2015.

Chapter 9:
How you Heal - Acupuncture, Herbal Therapy, Bodywork & Detoxification

Giménez G. et al. Cytotoxic effect of the pentacyclic oxindole alkaloid mitraphylline isolated from Uncaria tomentosa bark on human Ewing's sarcoma and breast cancer cell lines. *Planta Med.* 2010 Feb;76(2):133-6.

Bacher N. et al. Oxindole alkaloids from Uncaria tomentosa induce apoptosis in proliferating, G0/G1-arrested and bcl-2-expressing acute lymphoblastic leukaemia cells. *Br J Haematol.* 2006 Mar;132(5):615-22.

Pilarski R. et al. Antiproliferative activity of various Uncaria tomentosa preparations on HL-60 promyelocytic leukemia cells. *Pharmacol Rep.* 2007 Sep-Oct;59(5):565-72.

Riva L. et al. The antiproliferative effects of Uncaria tomentosa extracts and fractions on the growth of breast cancer cell line. *Anticancer Res.* 2001 Jul-Aug;21(4A):2457-61.

Dreifuss AA. et al. Uncaria tomentosa exerts extensive anti-neoplastic effects against the Walker-256 tumour by modulating oxidative stress and not by alkaloid activity. *PLoS One.* 2013;8(2):e54618.

de Paula LC. et al. Uncaria tomentosa (cat's claw) improves quality of life in patients with advanced solid tumors. *J Altern Complement Med.* 2015 Jan;21(1):22-30.

Tsai YL. et al. Cytotoxic effects of Echinacea purpurea flower extracts and cichoric acid on human colon cancer cells through induction of apoptosis. *J Ethnopharmacol.* 2012 Oct 11;143(3):914-9.

Luettig B. et al. Macrophage activation by the polysaccharide arabinogalactan isolated from plant cell cultures of Echinacea purpurea. *J Natl Cancer Inst.* 1989 May 3;81(9):669-75.

Joksić G. et al. Biological effects of Echinacea purpurea on human blood cells. *Arh Hig Rada Toksikol.* 2009 Jun;60(2):165-72.

Ninsontia C. et al. Silymarin selectively protects human renal cells from cisplatin-induced cell death. *Pharm Biol.* 2011 Oct;49(10):1082-90.

Post-White J. Ladas EJ. and Kelly KM. Advances in the use of milk thistle (Silybum marianum). *Integr Cancer Ther.* 2007 Jun;6(2):104-9.

Ramasamy K. and Agarwal R. Multitargeted therapy of cancer by silymarin. *Cancer Lett.* 2008 Oct 8; 269(2): 352–362.

Alessandro Federico A. Dallio M. and Loguercio C. Silymarin/Silybin and Chronic Liver Disease: A Marriage of Many Years. *Molecules* 2017, 22(2), 191.

Singh RP. and Agarwal R. Prostate cancer prevention by silibinin. *Curr Cancer Drug Targets.* 2004 Feb;4(1):1-11.

Katiyar SK. Silymarin and skin cancer prevention: anti-inflammatory, antioxidant and immunomodulatory effects (Review). Int J Oncol. 2005 Jan;26(1): 169-76.

Mastron JK. et al. Silymarin and hepatocellular carcinoma: a systematic, comprehensive, and critical review. *Anticancer Drugs.* 2015 Jun;26(5):475-86.

Csupor D. Csorba A. and Hohmann J. Recent advances in the analysis of flavonolignans of Silybum marianum. *J Pharm Biomed Anal.* 2016 Oct 25;130:301-317.

Kohno H. et al. Silymarin, a naturally occurring polyphenolic antioxidant flavonoid, inhibits azoxymethane-induced colon carcinogenesis in male F344 rats. *Int J Cancer.* 2002 Oct 10;101(5):461-8.

Fehér J. and Lengyel G. Silymarin in the Prevention and
    Treatment of Liver Diseases and Primary Liver Cancer.
    Current Pharmaceutical Biotechnology. 2012.13. 210-217.

Pardee AB. Li YZ. and Li CJ. Cancer therapy with beta-lapachone.
    Curr Cancer Drug Targets. 2002 Sep;2(3):227-42.

Balassiano IT. et al.. Demonstration of the lapachol as a potential drug for
    reducing cancer metastasis. *Oncol Rep.* 2005 Feb;13(2):329-33.

Kung HN. et al. Involvement of NO/cGMP signaling in the apoptotic and anti-
    angiogenic effects of beta-lapachone on endothelial cells in vitro.
    J Cell Physiol. 2007 May;211(2):522-32.

Babu MS. et al. Lapachol inhibits glycolysis in cancer cells by targeting pyruvate
    kinase M2. *PLoS One.* 2018; 13(2): e0191419.

Sunassee SN. et al. Cytotoxicity of lapachol, β-lapachone and related synthetic
    1,4-naphthoquinones against oesophageal cancer cells. *Eur J Med Chem.*
    2013 Apr;62:98-110.

Mahady GB. and Chadwick LR. Goldenseal (Hydrastis canadensis): Is There
    Enough Scientific Evidence to Support Safety and Efficacy? Nutrition in
    Clinical Care. 2001. 4(5): 243-249.

Lin H. et al. Inhibition of Gli/hedgehog signaling in prostate cancer cells by
    "cancer bush" Sutherlandia frutescens extract. Cell Biol Int. 2016 Feb;
    40(2): 131–142.

Skerman NB. Joubert AM and Cronjé MJ. The apoptosis inducing effects
    of Sutherlandia spp. extracts on an oesophageal cancer cell line.
    J Ethnopharmacol. 2011 Oct 11;137(3):1250-60.

Ntuli SSBN. Gelderblom WCA. and Katerere DR. The mutagenic and
    antimutagenic activity of Sutherlandia frutescens extracts and marker
    compounds. *BMC Complement Altern Med.* 2018 Mar 15;18(1):93.

van der Walt NB. Zakeri Z. and Cronjé MJ. The Induction of Apoptosis in
     A375 Malignant Melanoma Cells by Sutherlandia frutescens.
     Evid Based Complement Alternat Med. 2016;2016:4921067.

Chapter 10: Don't be a Victim of Your Genetics

World Cancer Research Fund and American Institute for Cancer Research.
     Continuous Update Project—eat whole grains, vegetables, fruits and
     beans. Access at
     https://www.wcrf.org/dietandcancer/recommendations/
     wholegrains-veg-fruit-beans

American Institute for Cancer Research. Foods that fight cancer—soy. Access at
     https://www.aicr.org/foods-that-fight-cancer/soy.html

Nishino H, et al. Cancer prevention by antioxidants. *Biofactors.*
     2004;22(1-4):57-61.

A Shenkin. Micronutrients in health and disease. *Postgrad Med J.*
     2006 Sep; 82(971): 559–567.

Chapter 12: Cannabis for Cancer

E. Joseph Brand and Zhongzhen Zhao. Cannabis in Chinese Medicine: Are
     Some Traditional Indications Referenced in Ancient Literature Related
     to Cannabinoids? *Front Pharmacol.* 2017; 8: 108.

National Cancer Institute. Cannabis and Cannabinoid. Physician Data Query,
     National Cancer Institute. Access at
     https://www.cancer.gov/about-cancer/treatment/cam/
     patient/cannabis-pdq

Grotenhermen F, Russo E, eds.: Cannabis and Cannabinoids: Pharmacology,
     Toxicology, and Therapeutic Potential. Binghamton, NY:
     The Haworth Press, 2002

Bifulco M, Laezza C, Pisanti S, et al.: Cannabinoids and cancer: pros and cons of an antitumour strategy. *Br J Pharmacol* 148 (2): 123-35, 2006.

Sánchez C, de Ceballos ML, Gomez del Pulgar T, et al.: Inhibition of glioma growth in vivo by selective activation of the CB(2) cannabinoid receptor. *Cancer Res* 61 (15): 5784-9, 2001.

Khasabova IA, Khasabov S, Paz J, et al.: Cannabinoid type-1 receptor reduces pain and neurotoxicity produced by chemotherapy. *J Neurosci* 32 (20): 7091-101, 2012.

Ward SJ, McAllister SD, Kawamura R, et al.: Cannabidiol inhibits paclitaxel-induced neuropathic pain through 5-HT(1A) receptors without diminishing nervous system function or chemotherapy efficacy. *Br J Pharmacol.* 171 (3): 636-45, 2014.

Richardson JD, Kilo S, Hargreaves KM: Cannabinoids reduce hyperalgesia and inflammation via interaction with peripheral CB1 receptors. *Pain.* 75 (1): 111-9, 1998.

Ibrahim MM, Porreca F, Lai J, et al.: CB2 cannabinoid receptor activation produces antinociception by stimulating peripheral release of endogenous opioids. *Proc Natl Acad Sci U S A* 102 (8): 3093-8, 2005.

Walker JM, Huang SM, Strangman NM, et al.: Pain modulation by release of the endogenous cannabinoid anandamide. *Proc Natl Acad Sci U S A* 96 (21): 12198-203, 1999.

Baker D, Pryce G, Giovannoni G, et al.: The therapeutic potential of cannabis. *Lancet Neurol* 2 (5): 291-8, 2003.

Rocha FC, Dos Santos Júnior JG, Stefano SC, et al.: Systematic review of the literature on clinical and experimental trials on the antitumor effects of cannabinoids in gliomas. *J Neurooncol* 116 (1): 11-24, 2014.

Sarfaraz S, Adhami VM, Syed DN, et al.: Cannabinoids for cancer treatment: progress and promise. *Cancer Res* 68 (2): 339-42, 2008.

Patsos HA, Hicks DJ, Greenhough A, et al.: Cannabinoids and cancer: potential for colorectal cancer therapy. *Biochem Soc Trans* 33 (Pt 4): 712-4, 2005.

Romano B, Borrelli F, Pagano E, et al.: Inhibition of colon carcinogenesis by a standardized Cannabis sativa extract with high content of cannabidiol. *Phytomedicine* 21 (5): 631-9, 2014.

McAllister SD, Murase R, Christian RT, et al.: Pathways mediating the effects of cannabidiol on the reduction of breast cancer cell proliferation, invasion, and metastasis. *Breast Cancer Res Treat.* 129 (1): 37-47, 2011.

Shrivastava A, Kuzontkoski PM, Groopman JE, et al.: Cannabidiol induces programmed cell death in breast cancer cells by coordinating the cross-talk between apoptosis and autophagy. *Mol Cancer Ther* 10 (7): 1161-72, 2011.

Cridge BJ, Rosengren RJ: Critical appraisal of the potential use of cannabinoids in cancer management. *Cancer Manag Res* 5: 301-13, 2013.

Blázquez C, Casanova ML, Planas A, et al.: Inhibition of tumor angiogenesis by cannabinoids. *FASEB J* 17 (3): 529-31, 2003.

Index

A

C

L

M